Stroke Hope
Stroke Awareness

by Daniel Bryan Jones

Copyright Statement

Publisher Statement

Stroke Hope Stroke Awareness is published by Daniel Bryan Jones.

Daniel Bryan Jones

Table of Contents

DISCLAIMER 6

FORWARD 7

REVIEWS 8

PREFACE 11

CHAPTER 1 12

CHAPTER 2 17

CHAPTER 3 31

CHAPTER 4 37

CHAPTER 5 46

CHAPTER 6 53

CHAPTER 7 59

CHAPTER 8 62

CHAPTER 9 69

CHAPTER 10 80

CHAPTER 11 86

CHAPTER 12 98

CHAPTER 13 101

CHAPTER 14 119

CHAPTER 15 127

ABOUT THE AUTHOR 134

Disclaimer

This publication is designed to provide general information regarding the subject matter covered.

Because each situation is different, the reader is advised to consult with his or her own advisor regarding that individual's specific situation.

Neither the author nor the publisher assume any responsibility for any errors or omissions, nor do they represent or warrant that the information, ideas, plans, actions, suggestions, and methods of operation contained herein is in all cases true, accurate, appropriate, or legal. It is the reader's responsibility to consult with his or her own advisor before putting any of the enclosed information, ideas, or practices into play. The author and the publisher specifically disclaim any liability resulting from the use or application of the information contained in this book, and the information is not intended to serve as legal advice related to individual situations. This book is a work of the author's experience and opinions only. Names, characters, places and incidents are either the product of the author's imagination or are used fictitiously. Any resemblance to actual persons, living or dead, or to actual events or locales is entirely coincidental.

Forward

What an interesting life. We all share the fact that we are mortal; different in that we have differing gifts and the same in that we live in a world that can sometimes be cruel. But through it all, there is love.

I have known Danny's parents for several decades but have only known Danny through them and mutual friends. From my once removed position, I have been impressed. He seemed to have the drive and intellect to lead a flourishing life.

But as sometimes happens, there was a cataclysmic life altering event. In light of the following, it seems Danny was perfectly equipped to handle and even flourish after surviving a near death experience:

God clearly is using Danny's exceptional drive to overcome adversity.

God has given him excellent care both medically and psychologically.

God has given him a superb wife who loves him and is hanging with him as not only a caregiver but best friend.

God is giving him a clear mind and insight as to his role in light of his new reality.

What a great example Danny's life is to others who experience the insecurity and fear resulting from great trauma. "Perfect love drives out fear" and clearly God is using Danny's experience to calm and redirect many who are enduring extreme difficulties.

William G. Billard

Elder, La Habra Hills Presbyterian Church
Past Board Chairman, Biola University
President retired, W.T. Billard, Inc.

Reviews

Review 1

February 14, 2013
Review for Danny Jones' book, "Stroke Hope Stroke Awareness".

I am privileged and pleased to have read the second book of Danny Jones, "Stroke Hope Stroke Awareness—Guide to Stroke Awareness." His book combines information with inspiration, fact with feelings, and reality with resources. It has proved to be great follow up to his first book, "God's Work", and I am certain that it will be an energetic launching for a Stroke Awareness series.

Danny writes clearly and methodically, inserting personal stories when appropriate, and providing a practical guideline for individuals and families who desire to learn about Stroke Awareness.

It promises to be a beneficial resource for anyone dealing with Stroke issues, whether personal or for a family member.

David A Eastis, MA in Theology, CTEC, business owner, Instructor/Teacher

••••••••••

Review 2

February 22, 2013
My review of "Stroke Hope Stroke Awareness" follows:
Title: Stroke Hope Stroke Awareness
Author: Daniel Bryan Jones
First Printing: June 2013
"Stroke Hope Stroke Awareness" is a breakthrough book.

It is perhaps the most useful self-help book I have ever read. Danny has been able to convey in a readable, well organized, and insightful way the challenges facing those recovering from a stroke, their caregivers, and family. If only I had access to this information, prior to two of my family suffering strokes, it would have so much easier to understand and help.

It will make a difference in the lives of all those touched by this tragedy.

Randall Jones, Sr. VP, GCT, retired.

•••••••••••

Review 3

Danny's follow-up to God's Work gives you an intimate tour into the world of strokes through education and anecdote. It's quite unique that Danny's research is written in conjunction with his own experience, having lived through a massive stroke in 2006. His firsthand account details his own tribulations, but also draws heavily on the vast knowledge he acquired from working with doctors and providers at one of the world's leading stroke recovery centers.

What makes Stroke Hope shine as something beyond that of just a valuable resource and insightful read is Danny's charisma — you can feel at ease while reading. He writes not to the academic community but to where his message is truly needed: the everyday man and woman. Most of us have a vague concept of what a stroke is, but how many of us would know the proper way to react if it occurred to a loved one right before our eyes? How about the critical steps taken immediately after and into recovery? Danny addresses it all, and more, while keeping it interesting and matter of fact.

The first volume of Stroke Hope may primarily deal with raising awareness, but it actually goes beyond that as it provides motivational guidance and spiritual assurance for those affected by strokes. Strokes may be damaging, but following the notes provided in the book can potentially lead to a recovery once thought impossible just a few decades ago.

Danny details the most efficient methods for recovery from his own experience, and there's much to be said about the value of experience when combined with research. In the end you gain much more than a glimpse into the realm of strokes, but rather a comprehensive understanding on how to deal, cope, and recover if the event ever happens to you or someone you know.

By James P. Goatcher

Preface

I was one of the lucky ones. I was able to have access to world-class cutting edge stroke post stroke care following my massive stroke in 2006. I spent over a year as an inpatient, first in a modern state of the art hospital, then at a world renowned brain injury facility. I was able to participate in daily therapy that was cutting edge at the time and only available to a select few stroke survivors.

In writing this book, I have drawn on my personal experiences in stroke rehab and recovery. I have read and researched everything I could find on the subject of stroke recovery and have spent hundreds of thousands of dollars to try to regain my health. Until you have lived through the highs and lows directly related to stroke and stroke recovery, you will never know what it is like to have suffered a significant stroke. In writing this book I have come full circle; and through adversity have come to realize that my stroke was not a punishment by God but a precious gift I could have never received unless I had it.

Danny Jones
Author/Writer Stroke Ambassador for American Heart and Stroke Assn.

Chapter 1

What is Aphasia?

What is aphasia?

Aphasia impairs the ability to speak and understand others, and most people with aphasia experience difficulty reading and writing.

What causes aphasia?

The ccrg St. Jude group for aphasia outreach: language impairment — or aphasia — occurs in more than a third of people who survive a stroke on the left side of their brain. Many recover within a few months after the stroke, but up to 60% still have language impairments more than six months after a stroke — a condition known as chronic aphasia.

"Usually patients in the chronic stage of aphasia receive about two hours of therapy a week over the course of a year, but we found that it is better to give the therapy within a shorter period of time," say researchers. Intense and frequent speech therapy early on seems to be what the experts agree on for aphasia treatment, for best results.

As many as 40% of all stroke survivors will develop some form of aphasia. Other causes for aphasia may be head trauma, brain tumor, and other brain injuries. Although aphasia is relatively unknown, more than 100,000 people acquire aphasia in the U.S. every year. Although aphasia is most common in older people, it can occur in all nationalities, and ages. Most people who experience aphasia will also experience paralysis or weakness of the right leg or arm or both.

Returning to work with aphasia can be difficult because most jobs require speech and language skills. If you or a loved one has aphasia, you may need to find new employment. Survivors who have experienced mild or moderate aphasia may be able to return to work full or part time. If you or a loved one is having problems speaking or understanding language, you will need to be evaluated by a speech therapist or be checked out by your rehab doctor.

Not all types of aphasia are alike.

Some people who have aphasia may have trouble speaking or may have lost the ability to form sentences.

* Others who suffer from aphasia may not be able to follow a conversation.

* They might know what they want to say but are not able to put the words together to form a coherent sentence.

* With mild forms of aphasia, you may not be able to notice it unless you know what to look for.

* In some cases of aphasia, the stroke survivor may have difficulty in speaking, writing, reading, or listening.

* Symptoms of aphasia vary widely from case to case. But most survivors with aphasia have some problems with communication. Similar to paralysis in the body, aphasia paralyzes the speech center located in the left hemisphere of the survivor's brain. Unfortunately, if the aphasia lasts longer than 2 to 3 months, the chances for the stroke survivor's complete recovery from aphasia drops significantly.

* Early and intense speech therapy is extremely important for survivors who acquire aphasia. Recovery from aphasia is most times a slow process. Survivors may continue to improve over a period of years or even decades.

* Although survivors with a aphasia may have difficulty finding the right words and retrieving thoughts, most times the survivor's intelligent is fully intact. Unlike Alzheimer's disease, it is the survivor's ability to access speech, ideas, and words through language that is the problem.

These problems with language skills may lead people to unmistakably assume that survivors suffering with aphasia are mentally ill or even retarded.

Aphasia is divided into four categories:

1. Expressive aphasia. These people have problems communicating with speech and writing. The survivor will

know what they want to say, but will not be able to find the words they want to say or write.

2. Receptive aphasia. This kind of aphasia causes the survivor to have difficulty understanding spoken or written language. They can see and hear the words, but cannot make sense of the spoken or written words.

3. Amnesia aphasia. This is the least severe type of aphasia. People with amnesia aphasia will still have trouble using the correct names for important events, people, places, or names for certain objects.

4. Global aphasia. Global aphasia is the most severe type of aphasia. This type of aphasia is caused by severe and extensive brain injury to the left side of the brain and the language center. Survivors with global aphasia may lose most of their ability to speak, and express language and writing skills. Most will be unable to speak, understand speech, or read and write.

There have been cases of patients with aphasia who have recovered completely without any treatment, although this should not be expected. Survivors who have aphasia should start speech and language therapy as soon as possible after being diagnosed with an aphasia disorder. Language therapy and work with a speech pathologist is highly recommended. Early and intense speech and language therapy has shown to be beneficial for stroke survivors who suffer from aphasia. The outcome of aphasia differs from case to case because of the wide range of aphasia conditions. Younger survivors and people who have suffered less severe brain injury tend to recover better and faster. Also where in the brain the brain injury occurred is also an important factor to the severity of the aphasia. Most aphasia patients tend to recover the ability to understand language comprehension better than they do in expressing their thoughts and language and writing skills.

Communicating with survivors who have aphasia: aphasia may impair the survivor from being able to communicate by speech, writing, or gestures. They may be unable to understand speech, gesture, or writings. Aphasia changes the way the survivor will communicate with family, friends, and coworkers.

The do's and dont's of communicating with survivors with aphasia:

1. Make sure you have the survivor's attention before trying to communicate with them.

2. Eliminate background noise. Turn off television and radio. Try to have a quiet place to communicate in.

3. Speak slowly and simplify your speech and sentence structure. You do not need to raise your voice, but speak clearly and emphasize the key words.

4. Introduce and encourage other kinds of communication as well as facial expressions.

* Make direct eye contact.

* Use writing, drawing, and yes and no responses.

* Use facial and hand gestures.

5. Do not be in a hurry or try to rush the survivor. Give them time to respond, and do not finish their sentences for them.

6. Do not criticize or correct the survivor. Instead, praise them when they attempt to talk and communicate. Do not expect them to pronounce every word correctly or perfectly.

7. Use speech, visual aids, and gestures. Repeat words or sentences as needed, and do not be overly protective.

8. Continue with normal activities. Try not to shield a survivor with aphasia, but include them in group conversation and decision-making when possible. Keep them informed of their care and mental and physical condition.

The types of aphasia:

1. Global aphasia: this type of aphasia is the most severe of all the types of aphasia. These survivors can only produce a few recognizable words and will only be able to understand little to no spoken words or language. Survivors with global aphasia usually cannot read or write. Global aphasia may occur immediately after stroke and improve rapidly if the

damage to the brain is not extensive.

2. Broca's aphasia, or more commonly known as non-fluent aphasia is when this survivor's speech is severely limited to mostly unrecognizable utterances of less than four words. Survivors with broca's aphasia often understand speech fairly well and may be able to read some but may not be able to write or draw.

3. Mixed non-fluent aphasia: this type of aphasia is when the patient has a sparse and effort filled speech. The survivor will remain limited in their comprehension of speech and will most likely be unable to read or write beyond an elementary level.

4. Wernicke's aphasia :(fluent-aphasia) is when the patient has trouble grasping the meaning of the spoken word but will be able to produce well connected speech. Hence the name "fluent-aphasia". With this form of aphasia reading and writing can often be severely compromised.

5. Anomic aphasia: is when the person with aphasia may know what they want to say or write but cannot find the words to express themselves. They may understand speech well and even understand what they are reading but can have difficulty responding in the spoken or written word.

Aphasia will occur in more than a third of all stroke survivors who have had a stroke on the left side of their brain. A full 60% of these aphasic survivors will continue to have chronic aphasia up to or exceeding six months following their stroke. Researchers say these aphasia suffers should have at least two hours of speech and language therapy a week, or more when possible.

Chapter 2

Benefits of Pet Ownership

Low energy pets like fish, cats, and other caged pets may be a better choice than dogs. Walking a dog is inherently dangerous. Four to six foot long leashes are best. Ten foot long leads are an accident waiting to happen. The use of self-feeding and watering bowls work quite well, house broken dogs and cats are a must. Puppies are out. One to two year old dogs are best. Old dogs are set in their ways and harder to acclimate.

Take your time choosing a rescue animal; they are hard to give back once you bring them home to the family. Ask yourself, do you need another thing in your life to take care of? Your stroke recovery should be your first priority and will be enough for most survivors.

A Good rule of thumb: small dog—small mess; big dog—big mess. Ten to fifteen lbs should be the cutoff.

Walking a dog can be hard enough without having to care for and clean up after it full time.

When dogs get spooked or scared they will run around you. They will wrap the leash around your legs and you're down before you know it. You cannot afford any falls. Another head injury and you might spend the rest of your life in a hospital. If you have to walk your dog, try to have someone go with you so you can hand the lead off to them if you get in trouble. Short leads of 4' to 6' in length should be the max.

When out for a walk in the park or neighborhood it's just a matter of time that you will come across someone walking their dog, and they always want to come up and let their dog sniff yours. If their dog is not friendly or your dog is aggressive you could have a dog fight on your hands.

Really? Don't you have more important things to work on

than taking care of a pet? Think about it again next year, if it still sounds like a good idea, then there will still be stray animals looking for a good home. There are lots of websites for pets that need a good home. Almost every breed of dog has a rescue website. I will expand later in this article. Rescue animals need rescuing for a reason.

Unlike a car, there is not always up to date information on all the animals offered for sale or adoption. Many have been abused or have matured with little training.

Puppies are always tough no matter what and require lots of care and training. Older dogs can be stubborn and hard to handle. They may be aggressive toward small children.

Always use caution in bringing a dog into the home, especially if young children are present. Find a neutral place to introduce a prospective pet to young children, and always make it clear that if the animal does not work out for any reason you reserve the right to return it for a full refund. Good luck, and use due diligence when selecting your next pet.

I have owned fifteen dogs in my lifetime and I don't think I have ever had any luck with a dog from the pound. In saying that I have to also tell you that many years ago I bought a "Scottie" on the spur of the moment for my daughter's birthday. Remember if you have kids and they get a pet it is most likely you or your spouse that will end up caring for it. The Scottie had been abused and would urinate every time you went to pet it. It was never right and I did not have a prior agreement to return it for a refund of the $350 I had spent on it. Their position was "buyers beware" and I or my daughter had done something to have caused the condition. Always and for any pet you adopt or purchase insist on a money back guarantee or a no fault" return agreement in writing with a termination date on the agreement.

Now for some good news: if you will take the time and have an open mind to a new idea. A pet can be a rewarding experience. There are literally hundreds of options you can choose from. Dogs and cats can be adopted for $25-$50 for cats and $100-$200 for dogs. This fee covers spay and neutering and other required shots. With some help from a friend or family member a couple times a week or even a paid service to walk and help with other pet needs you should be able to manage pet ownership. Fish, harmless snakes, turtles, and small gerbils can also be fun.

Some Benefits for Pet Ownership:

* Something to give you unconditional love and will always be there for you.

* Will help to increase exercise and activity levels and cause you to be playful.

* Pet ownership is known to reduce loneliness and stress levels.

* Pet ownership is thought to help increase new and expanded social interaction.

* There are many physical and mental benefits to pet ownership.

* Seniors who have regular interactions with a pet will have 30% fewer doctor visits than their counter parts who do not interact with a pet.

* Caring for a pet can help to raise self-esteem and will give you something to care for and love. Pet ownership may help to stave off boredom from being confined to a home or apartment.

* Studies show that in general pet owners have lower blood pressure, stress, and cholesterol levels than their non-pet owner counterparts and may put them at a reduced risk of heart attack and stroke.

* Dog owners are known to exercise more than non-owners of dogs. Playing with a kitten can also be helpful in getting needed exercise.

* Pet owners are thought to have less depression and be less likely to suffer from loneliness and isolation than non-pet owners.

* Pet ownership has been proven to improve one's social skills.

* Pet ownership has proven to reduce the number of doctor visits in elderly survivors.

* Pets help to ease the sense of loss in older survivors who have lost a spouse or loved one; they are less likely to experience health deterioration if they are attached to a pet.

* Pet owners report less headaches and less difficulty in sleeping.

Many of these benefits of pet ownership are attributed directly to the basic human need for being touched. Studies have shown that merely holding or petting a pet can calm, sooth, and help to reduced anxiety and stress in humans who are experiencing high stress levels in their lives. Even watching a fish swim in a fish bowl has shown to lower heart rate and reduce muscle tension in the body.

Pets that stimulate activity and exercise may reduce your risk of obesity, lower the chance of becoming depressed, and increase social interaction.

Pets Help the Survivor to Make
Healthy Lifestyle Changes by:

* By having to care for a pet you may decrease the chance of developing depression and anxiety disorders.

* Helping the survivor to get a routine by walking, feeding or other needed care, no matter what mood you are in. Structure and routine are known to be beneficial for the stroke survivor's recovery, both mental and physical.

* Just having to get out of bed and dress every day to care for something that is dependent on us is good for the moral.

The basic need for touch and being loved can be fulfilled by petting a cat or snuggling with a puppy. These activities can reduce your chances of stress related ailments.

Pet ownership offers you a new way to get needed exercise. Add these activities to your regular training regimen.

Walking a dog around the block; or chasing a kitten or bunny around the yard can give you an added aerobic exercise.

I know when I was walking my rescue dog "Moony" I would see the same folks every day out walking their dogs. Some of them I became friendly with in time and shared small talk with them when we would cross paths. We would stop and talk together to share current affairs and news about our dogs.

Owning a pet will give you something in common with people who own similar animals. There are events put on you can attend by the different pet associations, where you can get information on new care products for your particular pet and also have the opportunity to meet and make new and lasting friendships. Dogs, cats, reptiles, horses, and all kinds of farm animals have groups you can join.

Following a stroke, survivors may become isolated and lonely. These conditions can put you at an increased risk of becoming depressed. Pet ownership may help to reduce this risk by keeping the survivor busy and focused on something other than themselves.

Despair, loneliness, and depression can all follow a significant stroke, ESPECIALLY when brain injury has been suffered.

Finding the Right Pet for You:

Studies have shown that stroke survivors who own and care for a pet are more likely to be more secure, happier, and independent than non-pet owners.

Choosing the right pet for your lifestyle and taking in account for any physical limitations can be important to both you and your prospective pet.

For instance, if you are forced to spend most of your time indoors, you may want to look into pets that do not need to be out of doors a lot, like farm animals and large bread dogs. Large dogs that need a lot of exercise can suffer when locked up inside for days on end. You can consider instead maybe a small dog or kitten. Watching or caring for fish or reptiles may be a better choice for your present situation, and when your situation changes you can reconsider a different pet choice.

Birds do well indoors. Parrots and cockatoos can be good company and relate well to humans.

If you are active and spend time outdoors, you may want to consider dog ownership. Walking or running a dog can be an excellent source of daily exercise that can help to control excess body weight, improve cardiovascular health, and help reduce the risk for depression and anxiety disorder.

When Bringing a New Pet into the Home:

* Some dogs do not do well with children, especially older animals. It's best to raise dogs and children together when possible. Puppies and kittens will usually be safe around small children — take it slow and have close supervision of all new pets introduced to the family home.

Pets and Children:

* Delicate pets need to be handled with care and may need to be kept out of the reach of small children.

* Large and active dogs can accidentally knock a small child to the ground and cause them injury.

* Always do a pet inventory of existing pets in the home before bringing a new pet into the home. For instance, if you have cats in the home, they may not mix well when bringing a dog into the home, while some dogs can be possessive and not want to share you with a new arrival.

Cats can be dangerous and lash out when spooked and scratch a child. Cat bites and scratches are potentially very dangerous and can turn septic if not treated immediately.

* Always choose pets that match your lifestyle. If you tend to be a "neat freak" a long hair un-housebroke puppy that

chews on everything may not be the right choice for you.

* Caged pets like fish, birds, and small gerbils may be a better fit for you.

* Consider where your new dog will spend most of its time. A new dog may dig holes in your yard or even destroy small trees and bushes. The urine of un-spayed female dogs will leave yellow patches in the lawn.

* Before making a commitment to bring a pet into your home keep in mind that many pets can live for many years. Once you become attached to them they can be hard to let go. Dogs and cats can live for 10-20 years. They will need daily care and may need expensive medical care and shots from time to time. There is no affordable health insurance for animals, and vets can cost as much as medical doctors. Birds and some reptiles like turtles can live for decades.

* Keep in mind that if you travel for work or vacation someone will need to care for your pets, and boarding can be expensive too.

Some Reasons for Not Wanting to Get a Pet:

* Not having time to care for a pet.

* Loss of a job or income.

* Living in a small home, apartment, or care facility.

* New or worsening disability or health concerns.

* Fear and increased risk of injury, being knocked down, or tripping over a pet.

* Issues with pet transportation—required trips to the vet or groomer.

* Adequate help with a new pet, concerns for being able to care properly for a pet.

Finding Help Caring
For a New Pet

* Vets, groomers, and trainers that will make house calls.

* Kennels that will pick up and return your pet for you.

* In-home sitters and walkers; they now have day care for dogs and will pick up and return pets for you.

* You can order food and pet supplies online and have it delivered to your home — many offer free shipping.

* Many shelters offer pets that are house broke and trained to live in an in-home environment. These pets are well suited for older survivors who are not able to keep up with a young animal.

If you rent, you should get in-writing permission and terms of pet ownership. For instance; you might have taken in a rescue dog from the county pound and have kept it a secret for three months, you fall in love with your new pet and spent hundreds of dollars getting the pet moved in, then have your landlord find out that you have an unapproved pet and demand that you remove the pet, or worse evict you for having it. Either way you would have been better off to have had permission first. I'm a realtor by trade and I will tell you that most property owners don't like pets in their rentals. Too much liability connected to pets.

Start small in whatever you decide on. Remember, little pet little mess — big pet big mess. And be sure to choose a pet you can get rid of if it becomes more than you can take care of. Remember you will get attached to small furry animals you spend time caring for.

"Moony" the rescue dog

Mooney: after returning home from the hospital and rehab facility I lived in for two years, I had started having thoughts. *A dog sounded fun*. I had owned dogs for most of my life. From my childhood until I burned out, after breeding

American Staffordshire terriers for ten years. From the day I put down my last pit bull in 1980 until my stroke now, at the thanksgiving holiday, did my wife June or I ever talk about getting another dog.

With me spending more time at home the thought of having a dog to keep me company seemed like it might be a good idea. And it might give an otherwise doomed dog another chance to get a good home. Most dogs in county animal shelters are destroyed in the first thirty days after they arrive. Some ten million animals every year nationwide.

I started my quest for a dog by dropping hints and feeling my wife out on the acquisition of a dog. It was clear from the very beginning what she thought. She did not think that a dog was anything I needed to get involved with. And she assured me that she did not desire to own a dog at this particular juncture in our lives. "Don't we have enough on our plates without keeping up with a dog?" What would we do when we wanted to travel?" she would ask me.

The weeks passed and I kept up the pressure up. I started looking online and would leave printouts of dogs ready to be adopted out on the coffee table—the orange county animal shelter was located a short drive from our home in Southern California.

By now, June knew that I had set my mind on getting a dog. I'm sure she was hoping I would be up to the task of being able to care for a dog. And it might even give me a sense of responsibility and also be of some company for me during the day.

The day would come on a Saturday morning right before thanksgiving holiday 2011. June and I made the fifteen minute drive to the animal shelter. I was carrying a printout of an eight pound Chihuahua named Moony. It said he was two years old. I had owned big dogs and knew big pets meant big messes. I also knew that younger than two years were the "puppy years" and older than three, a dog could be set in their ways and harder to train. After all, I had bred and raised dogs for over a quarter century.

We went into a Mobile home trailer set up to handle the process of adopting a pet. Dogs and cats. We waited in line with the others there that wanted to adopt a pet. When your number was called the woman behind the counter gave you paperwork that allowed you to go on the lot and look through the cages to find a pet you were interested in adopting.

We went to where the dogs were housed. The first cage in the first aisle we looked in was the chihuahua "Moony" all eight scrawny pounds of him. You could tell that living on the lam was not agreeing with him. He was very emaciated and looked dirty. If ever there was a dog needing to be rescued it was moony. After we found the dog we wanted, a face to face meeting with it would be arranged. We had to go back to the trailer and stand in line all over again until our new number was called by the woman behind the counter, which we now knew on a first name basis. We told her what dog we wanted to see, and she gave us another slip of paper and told us to go back by where the dog was and a handler would come and bring the dog we wanted to see to us. There was a small fenced in area about 30' square with a chair in the middle in which I sat. The handler lead moony up and down the pen, and when he came within an arm's length away from me I reached down and said his name and cradled him in the palm of my hand around his chest and lifted him and held him close. I knew Chihuahuas were skittish, but he never made a sound or tried to jump away from me.

He was the right age. They said he was two years old, but I think he was much younger; he was maybe a year old at best. Shelters stretch a puppy's age because it is easier to get them adopted. I had raised dogs professionally for years and I know a puppy when I see one.

Then we had to go again to the line I was getting tired of standing in. After June and I discussed it, I told the young woman behind the counter that we would adopt moony. She then said it would be $165 for the neuter and the minimum shots they gave the dogs before releasing them. It also covered one year dog license. And because it was the thanksgiving holiday it could take five days instead of the usual three for his release.

It ended up taking the five. We had gone to Petco and purchased some things a new dog would need. We soon picked him up, where they discharged the dogs, and put the collar and leash on him and lead him to the car to bring him home.

I have made a list of the startup costs you should expect to be spending to start off with, your costs may vary.

Getting dog spayed or neutered and shots and license fee $165

Food and water bowels $75

Lead and collar $50

Dog bed $40

Doggy training $110

Chew toys and other toys $60

Monthly grooming $55

Vet and shots $150

My startup costs for a rescue dog $705

For a free dog.

Moony coming home:

He was needy from the start. All that moony wanted to do was to be next to me. I think he thought it was his job to be glued to my right hip.

When we took him out into the neighborhood for a walk or down to the little park in our neighborhood, if moony saw or even smelled another dog in the area he would start pulling with his entire might against his leash. If he got the chance, he would attack another dog every time. He even tried to bite a 100lb. Pit bull at the obedience school I took him to. It was clear from the start that he was too young to be ready for any advanced training. I asked for, and they refunded the cost of the obedience school in a credit for future purchases — we used the credit for food and grooming.

From Moony's very first day he was determined that he be allowed to be a house dog. The first house dog I had owned in my lifetime.

He slept at the foot of my bed with me. He liked to stay covered with a small blanket lying close enough to me to feel me.

Then all day from the time we went down to the couch to watch the morning news and having my coffee he stayed curled up next to me. From then till we went back up or June brought him up for the night. I figured that he spent conservatively twenty hours a day stuck to me at the right hip.

He soon started going down when he heard June my wife come in from a day at work. He would then go and be needy with her for hours until she brought him up to me for the night, where he would stay under the covers till I got up the next morning to do it all over again.

There was something wrong with him from the start. He was very skittish and would nip at me when he was startled. He continued to attack any dogs he could get close to. This went on for three to four months.

One morning as we were getting ready to go downstairs to start the day. He was extra nervous and jumpy. He jumped down off the bed and ran down the hall into my wife's room. He had done it before looking for her. I went downstairs and waited for him to follow just like every other morning since he had been with us.

After a while I called out for him to come. He usually did come. After an hour or so of calling his name every fifteen minutes, I went upstairs to find him hiding in the back of June's walk in closet among her pairs of shoes.

I called for him to come out to me, and when he didn't I thought that this strange behavior for our new dog Moony.

I wanted him to come downstairs where I could watch him. He would still wet the carpet when he wasn't being supervised. When he refused to come out of June's closet I stepped in and reached in to grab him by the nap of his the neck like a mother dog would do when moving her pups around.

When I grabbed him he turned on me and bit me by my hand and fingers of my right hand. Shocked and startled from the attack, I fell backwards almost braining myself on the doorjamb. He would also run around my legs when walking causing me to have fallen several times before. My hand was severely bitten and I would need first aid for the bite.

So after talking to June by phone from her work we decided we could not keep a dog that would bite someone. And we would not take the chance that he would get spooked by one of the grandkids and bite them in the face.

I called my mother in-law and asked her if she would give me a ride to the county animal shelter to return him.

He had bitten me badly enough to make me bleed from the wounds to the three fingers of my right hand.

I had decided not to tell them at the animal shelter that moony had bitten anyone and to give him another chance of someone adopting him again. He was a pretty little dog. He had filled out from the regular meals he got while staying with us.

When the young woman running the intake shed had me sign the return form she saw the wounds to my right hand. She asked me point blank, "Did he do that"?

I didn't feel like lying for him and thought it not fair to let someone else get bitten.

She told me then that he would have to be put down as a biter and that after the first attack they were more likely to bite someone again. My grandmother had a little Chihuahua in Texas that kept my brother Joe and I afraid from the time we got to grandma and grandpas house till we left. It was a classical 'ankle bitter'.

A handler came and took the lead from my ma's hand and led him away. I know he had to be remembering all the sounds and smells. He had been at the animal shelter for thirty days when June and I rescued him.

The moral to my story is an easy one. Do not get in a hurry; Do your due diligence and background check on any animal you plan to adopt. There is always a reason why they are there in the first place. You can always take them back if it doesn't work out for you or the pet. Figure out your costs, and if the breed is going to fit within your surroundings.

After years of raising dogs I will assure you that keeping animals is a lot of work.

Although I included animal shelter information, I should have known better than to invest time and money into a shelter animal. I cannot in good conscience recommend a dog from the "pound". Shelter dogs are there most times for a reason. They can be very needy, hard to leave alone, hard to house break, and aggressive towards children.

I know some people do not care for cats, but they may be a better choice and a lot less work than a dog.

Chapter 3

Brian Injury,
TBI and Plasticity

Brain injury is said to be any change to the brain that affects someone's behavior, emotions, or physical well-being. Brain injuries may be caused at birth,

Brain injuries may be either traumatic or non-traumatic in nature.

Traumatic brain injury can be a not limited to:

* Motor vehicle accidents.

* Loss of consciousness.

* Military attacks or bomb blast.

* Gunshot or other violence.

Loss of consciousness, open head wound, or skull fracture does not always result in dramatic brain injury.

Non traumatic brain injury:

* Lack of blood flow or oxygen to the brain.

* Injuries at birth or other illness like cancer.

* Stroke is the leading cause for non-traumatic brain injury.

* Some invasive surgeries.

Brain injury: brain injury is not an event or an outcome. It is the start of a misdiagnosed, misunderstood, under-funded neurological disease. Individuals who sustain brain injuries must have timely access to expert trauma care, specialized rehabilitation, lifelong disease management, and individualized services and supports in order to live healthy, independent and satisfying lives.

The brain injury association of America (BIAA) is the voice of brain injury. They are dedicated to increasing access to quality health care and raising awareness and understanding of brain injury through advocacy, education, and research. With a nationwide network of state affiliates, local chapters, and support groups, they provide help, hope, and healing for individuals who live with brain injury, their families, and the professionals who serve them.

Brain injury warning signs: **seek medical attention if you are experiencing any of these:**

* **Numbness**
* **Excessive drowsiness**
* **Severe headache**
* **Weakness in your arms or legs**
* **Dizziness or loss of vision**
* **Slurred speech**
* **Loss of consciousness**
* **Vomiting**

Traumatic brain injury (tbi), also known as **intracranial injury,** occurs when an external force traumatically injures the brain. Tbi can be classified based on severity, mechanism (closed or penetrating head injury), or other features (e.g., occurring in a specific location or over a widespread area). Head injury usually refers to tbi, but is a broader category because it can involve damage to structures other than the brain, such as the scalp and skull.

Tbi is a major cause of death and disability worldwide, especially in children and young adults. Causes include falls, vehicle accidents, and violence. Prevention measures include use of technology to protect those suffering from automobile accidents, such as seat belts and sports or motorcycle helmets, as well as efforts to reduce the number of automobile accidents, such as safety education programs and enforcement of traffic laws.

Brain trauma can be caused by a direct impact or by acceleration alone. In addition to the damage caused at the moment of injury, brain trauma causes secondary injury, a variety of events that take place in the minutes and days following the injury. These processes, which include alterations in cerebral blood flow and the pressure within the skull, contribute substantially to the damage from the initial injury.

Behavioral changes caused by stroke may vary and be the direct result to the strokes severity and where in the brain the stroke was located. Strokes are most common in the cerebral cortex, which has two hemispheres

1. The right hemisphere which controls emotions, sense of body position, relative location, and non-verbal communication.

2. The left hemisphere which controls the right side of the body. The brain's language center. The left hemisphere is also responsible for one's analytical thinking and comprehension. The chronic loss of balance is also a symptom of right hemisphere brain injury.

Right-brain injury: survivors who experience damage to the right side of the brain may not be aware to the extent that they are impaired. Many times the stroke survivor with right-brain injury may feel that they are able to perform the same tasks as they could before their stroke. This type of brain injury may leave the survivor with poor judgment, short-term memory loss, a short attention span, and in some cases they may be emotionally unstable. Stroke survivors who have suffered right brain injury may have trouble performing simple tasks that can make others see them as being unmotivated, dependent on others, confused, and even uncooperative in some cases. Not until the survivor is fully aware of their limitations due to a right-brain injury can they or their caregiver start to train them to be safe in their potentially dangerous environments. Right side brain injured survivors need to have a safe environment to live in. free of trip and other hazards.

Survivors who have experienced right side brain injury often have loss of vision on their left side peripheral vision. It is important that they learn to be able to scan their vision from side to side. With "left neglect", remember that the affected part of your body is still a part of you. Ask people when they enter a room that you are occupying to enter the room on the side that your vision is best. Ask them to approach you on your right side and speak to you as they enter. This will allow you to know when someone is entering the room. Be sure to rub or touch your affected left side often and ask family members to do it also. It is important that in the first days following your stroke that you have stimulation to those weak parts of your body that have stopped moving and may have become paralyzed due to a stroke.

Be sure to ask for help when you need it — going in alone may cause you undue injury. Trying to do jobs, like changing light bulbs, hanging Christmas lights, and changing the batteries in the smoke detectors should be avoided. Getting on a ladder for any reason with balance issues is foolhardy at best. Ask caregivers to place items that you might need on your right side if you're left side vision is impaired. A calm uncluttered environment is preferred for survivors with right side brain injury.

Eliminate all clutter and distractions, including any trip and fall risks like loose rugs, toys, and pets in the home. Right side brain injury can affect the survivor's depth perception and limits vision to the left peripheral and all vision on the left side. Furniture and other items with sharp edges found in the home should be stored away or clearly marked. Some survivors with right brain injury may have some speech or other communication difficulties due to the weakness in the facial muscles. Many will have varying degrees of Bell's palsy. Still a smaller percentage of right brain survivors can have difficulty interacting normally due to problems with thinking clearly and confusion. For speech and language problems, a speech therapist should be contacted early following a stroke.

Left Side Brain Injury:

Stroke survivors who have suffered a left side brain injury may experience paralysis to their right side, personality change, and difficulty communicating with both the spoken and written word. They may know what they want to say or write but will be unable to find the words to express themselves. Survivors with left side brain injury often behave in a disorganized, compulsive, or an over cautious manner. They may also be slow to respond to questions, or take action when it is not required.

Care Givers Should
Help the Survivor by:

It is important for the caregiver to establish daily routines and schedules. These activities will need to be carefully planned around any limitations the survivor with a left side brain injury is experiencing. Be careful not to cause fatigue that can lead to exhaustion. This type of brain injury will make the survivor susceptible to fatigue and cause them to tire more easily. If they are not careful, this fatigue or exhaustion can slow the survivor's recovery. Be patient when communicating with the survivor and do not rush them to answer or respond to questions. Also do not try to finish their sentences for them. Speak to the survivor in a normal tone; the confusion they are experiencing is in the brain, but they can most times hear you fine. Give feedback and use other forms of communicating. Hand gestures, facial cues, and writing or drawing. It is helpful to use yes and no questions when speaking with the survivor who has a left side brain injury.

Brain plasisticty neuroplasticity
My thoughts and experience with brain injury after stroke:
I will start with the misconception about the so called 'crossover theory' in my humble opinion it is a wives' tale. An utter misunderstanding of brain plasticity.

Symptoms for brain injury:
* Headache.
* Loss of coordination and balance.
* Trouble moving arms or legs normally.

* Loss of bladder or bowel control.

* Onset of seizures.

* Blurred or loss of vision in one or both eyes.

* Slurred speech and or difficulty swallowing.

* Changes of sleep patterns.

After my stroke in 2006, to this day in late 2012 i still have all eight of these symptoms on my left side. Brain injury never heals — what you have six months following your stroke is most likely what you will have the rest of your life barring any miracle. Returns and changes in these early symptoms usually happen in the first hours, days, or weeks and months following a stroke.

Other functional and changes in emotions from brain injury may include:

* Loss of short-term memory and being unable to remember ongoing conversations.

* Limited or loss of attention span.

* Unable to convey what you are thinking to others. Loss of the ability to form a coherent sentence.

* Confusion.

* Depression. Half of all stroke survivors will suffer from depression and or anxiety within one year following their stroke.

* Unable to concentrate, reason, to be logical, and loss of focus.

* Mood swings brought on by stress or anxiety.

Chapter 4

Caregivers, they do
God's Work in a Survivor's Life

If you are taking on the role of a primary caregiver for a stroke survivor, you will be taking on many new and varying responsibilities. Be prepared to deal with the stress that will surely come with these new and ever changing commitments. If you are a spouse or family member, it may help to share your concerns with other family members; if the stress becomes too much, you may need to turn the care of the survivor over to the professionals who deal with ongoing care giving.

If the care giving responsibilities fall too heavily on one person, the duties of care giving can become extremely stressful or even overwhelming. Sometimes when family does get involved in the care giving process, conflicts can break out over care giving issues, like finances and other duties.

Learning to deal with new and increasing stress is important for keeping yourself healthy while caring for your loved one. Remember that you also need understanding and a time for rest too.

Making and Keeping Appointments:

After your loved one has returned home from the hospital or rehab facility they will need to have regular doctor and rehab appointments, maybe for years. These appointments are important in monitoring the survivor's ability to use the new skills they have gained in their recovery following the stroke. It is equally important for the survivor's many doctors and therapists to determine how well they are adjusting to the many physical and mental changes brought on by their recent stroke.

Family members can help their loved one by providing encouragement, celebrating improvements, and letting the survivor do as much as possible independently. Caregivers and other family and friends can reassure stroke survivors that they are wanted, needed, and important to them.

Providing care for a loved one after stroke can be an extremely rewarding experience. At the same time, it can be stressful and frustrating when you are suddenly thrust into the position of caregiver without warning. The information here will help you take care of not only the stroke survivor in your life, but yourself.

The first hours and days of the stroke survivor's recovery are the most important for at least two reasons:

1. I call it the golden hours. The longer you survive after a stroke the better the chance you have for survival. My doctor told my family that I would never live longer than the first three days following my stroke. That nobody lived through that massive of a stroke. Nobody.

2. What you do in the first days and the choices you make in regards to your recovery will set the course for the rest of your recovery. You have a limited time after brain injury and stroke, to return function to what is damaged and will return to normal. My bladder took six months of me being straight cathead every four hours around the clock. The urinary doctor elected for me to get the straight one time cath instead of a more permanent catheter and leg bag.

3. At first when I would go into the bathroom every morning to have a bowel movement, when I strained from the constipation I experienced from the opiates I took, I found I could squeeze a few drops of urine out. This went on for weeks slowly getting more urine to flow. I had family and friends praying for me—I knew that life on a leg bag would be harder, but you do what you have to. If you must use a permanent catheter so be it, you will learn to live with it.

4. Be careful not to overdue things and injure yourself. If it was sheer-will I would be running the Los Angeles marathon

this year.

5. The survivor's recovery is built on one building block to the next. It is good for him or her to stretch the limits from time to time. Getting tired often builds stamina, both mentally and physically. They will need endurance to keep building their recovery.

6. Stroke can be and is usually as much mental as physical.

What are Advocates, and do I need one? Without someone with you in the hospital after a stroke, you are last in line. Someone needs to make daily visits to check on your ongoing care. To check if you're getting showered, shaved, and fingernails and toe nails trimmed. They need to check to be sure you are eating regularly and order meals and make sure doctors are making their regular rounds and updating the survivor's condition. Also to make sure that therapies are scheduled and that you are going every day. The first days and the golden hours are very real; once they are past, you will never get to do them over again.

I think most hospitals have access to social workers but even then you need someone monitoring what's going on with the survivor's care and recovery.

Note to survivors:

Your caregivers will burnout and will do better if you try to help yourself as much as you are able. They get tired day in and day out. If you do not get a dog in the fight and take some control of your own recovery, they will tire of trying to motivate you. Just a word to the wise, if you don't try and help them and yourself, you run the risk of one day they stop coming.

I can't emphases strongly enough. It is important to compliment and acknowledge your caregivers often.

Whether they are friends helping out, family members, or a spouse or a paid trained professional aid everyone appreciates being complimented.

You need to be kind and complimentary with them in their dealings with you and your care. It is for the most part a difficult thankless job anyway.

I told a young woman one day while still at Casa Colina, "You know I'm a millionaire don't you?"

She replied, "Yes, I have heard that."

I then told her that I could not do her job for the money I made and I meant it.

You should treat your helpers with the respect and care that you would wish to be treated. It's a hard job, whoever has to do it.

I have found in my own dealings with caregivers that it is also important to do your best to assist in your care whenever you are able. To safely help a caregiver gives you the chance to see to what extent you are able to assist them and gives you the chance to practice the steps needed for recovery. It's one time you want to work someone out of a job.

Your independence will increase with time and hard work. Take your time, but be steady and try new things to see the extent of your ability to help in your personal care and recovery.

Others will notice your willingness to get involved in your own care and recovery. This will be seen by those helping you as a sign of recovery and that you are getting more independent.

If you get hardened, nasty, and argumentative, you run the real risk of your helpers burning out and up and quitting you.

I know as well as any how miserable it is to live as an invalid and handicapped. But caregivers are in some cases a must have commodity.

Toe and fingernails: Hospitals and care facilities will not cut finger and toe nails. From the very start you need to make frequent checks of the stroke survivor's nails

Toe nails: should be trimmed every month.

Finger nails: they grow more quickly and should be trimmed every two to three weeks at most.

A podiatrist should be hired when the survivor is going to

stay long term in a facility or hospital.

Safety first.

When first starting to care for a stroke survivor you need to stress, safety first. Falls injure more people in the United States every year than all other accidents combined. If your survivor has weakness in one or both arms or hands, they have no way to break a fall.

Some Steps to Avoid
Caregiver Burnout:

For many Americans, care giving is and will not be a short term arrangement but can last for decades. And in many cases the one being cared for will outlast the caregiver. In some instances aging parents will "guilt" their adult children into providing for their every need; by declining to accept outside help. They will tell them "you are to only one who can do what I expect out of a caregiver".

When you take on the caregiver role. Start by compiling three lists, detailing your commitments. Things that you should not be negotiable on:

1. Like your job, caring for your children, and things needed to run a household.

2. Paying bills, home maintenance, and shopping and cleaning.

3. "Me" time, time you use only for yourself. This time is important for recharging your batteries. You might have lunch with a friend, read, or just rest in a quiet place.

This time alone is critical in avoiding caregiver burnout and should be for at least seven hours a week.

After compiling your lists, determine what time is left over for care giving. With this time you will decide the most important things your loved one needs assistance with, and things you are able to help with.

Now Make Another List:

1. The names of family and friends you can call on for help. The "Deacons" from your local church can be a good source of help—most people are glad to pitch in if they are only asked; all they can do is say in no.

2. For the ones who do say yes, find out the days and times they will be available to help and note it next to their name.

You will need help with getting to doctors' appointments, preparing meals, and other required chores.

3. Have a heart to heart talk with the loved one needing assistance. It is helpful to include the people who will be helping if possible, to discuss the survivor's true needs, and the one which will be helping and when.

At this meeting it is important for you to make your own commitments clear. Be firm on what you are able to commit to and don't back down. This will set the tempo for your care giving. If they become disappointed or argumentative, it might be a good time to discuss the possible need for outside help. Many aging adults will not accept the loss of independence and may not want to accept outside help, and at the same time they are working their adult child to death. Be understanding but firm.

4. Be careful not to become a maid or butler to the survivor and do not be afraid to request the survivor to get involved in their own care and recovery. Don't do things for them that they are able to do for themselves.

5. When a survivor gets angry and frustrated keep in mind it's usually not the caregiver but can be more about the loss of control, independence, and other changes they are going through, and the inability to accept those difficult changes.

6. Keep your eye on the ball; keep your personal needs in mind at all times. If you do not take care of yourself, you will soon lose the ability to take care of your loved one. If and

when you feel you're losing control and getting overwhelmed, you may need to seek outside help. You may need to solicit assistance from close friends or family. An excellent source for help can be from the deacons at your local church.

7. Make a list of the things the survivor can do safely for themselves, and you can add to the list as they become more independent with time.

8. Let go and let God. Do not feel guilty. There is no such thing as Superman. No one can fix everything that comes their way. Guilt is the number one cause for caregiver burn out.

9. SAFTY FIRST, for the caregiver and survivor alike. Survivors who have experienced brain injury often want to continue making decisions about their care long after they are capable of doing so.

10. Try not to take the survivor's anger and frustrations personally.

11. Post stroke caregivers and family members will play an important role throughout the survivor's post stroke recovery process. Caregivers and family members are mandatory for successful in-home care and often go unappreciated or properly thanked for their unselfish, consistent, and daily assistance for the stroke survivor.

Trying to care for a stroke survivor on an in-home basis can cause high levels of stress on an emotional and physical level, not to mention the disruption of employment and family life. Undue stress and worry can make care giving a very challenging proposition.

When properly done, family caregivers can assist the survivor in their positive post stroke recovery; however, they must take care not to let their own needs get neglected. You need to take care of yourself because if you get unhealthy, it may cause the one you are caring for to suffer also.

As is common in caregivers of Alzheimer's patients, also with stroke survivors, the one being cared for may outlive the caregiver in many cases.

If you find you are unable to financially care for a

survivor at home any longer, there may be state and federal help for stroke survivors who require twenty-four hour care. Consult with the survivor's doctors and inquire to what the chances of a full or partial recovery can be expected for them.

You may need to have a part time caregiver come to the home several times a week to help with the care of the stroke survivor. There are also in-home therapy companies that will visit your home to provide needed therapies following a stroke. Check with your insurance company and inquire to see the extent of coverage for post stroke care.

Care Givers and Family Members
May be required to assist
In the Following:

* Assist in driving to doctor's appointments, filling medications, and trips to exercise facilities.

* Help in paying bills and other financial matters.

* Arranging transportation for required appointments and other outings.

* Assistance in planning and organizing hobbies and travel.

* Facilitate the survivor's medical needs and be their advocate to obtain the best possible care from hospitals and insurance companies.

* Help in planning strategies for recovery, setting and carrying out routines, and managing the survivor's "care team".

* Assist the survivor in their daily activities, like personal care and hygiene.

* Provide mental and emotional support.

Caregivers, Family Members, Or Spouses Who Have to Cope With This Condition May Want to:

* Take care of yourself first. When you find yourself getting tired out either physically, mentally, or emotionally you may need to seek out professional care for yourself and the survivor if needed.

* Look for a support network, feeling alone can cause you to feel defeated and forgotten. You can go online to look for stroke caregiver support groups in your area.

* Understand that no one is perfect and it is understandable that you will make mistakes. Take it slow. You and the survivor you're are caring for will learn to cope together.

* Take regular breaks away from the stressful duties of care giving. Just like work, and it is work, you run the risk of burning out if you overdue it. If you allow your health to deteriorate, you will be of no use to either yourself or the survivor. Be sure to take time to rest yourself if you feel yourself becoming fatigued.

* When you feel yourself getting upset or irritated at the survivor you are caring for, it's time to step back and catch your breath. Explain your frustrations and be upfront and honest with them, and try not to let situations fester and spin out of control. The best time to address these feelings is the present—don't wait.

Chapter 5

Driving Again After Stroke

In most states there is a law that if you lose consciousness from any medical condition whether it be heart attack seizure or stroke, the D.M.V. is by law required to revoke your driver's license for an undetermined length of time.

For reinstatement of your driver's license you must prove you are medically fit to drive and pass a driver's test. You must also have a doctor sign off on your condition.

In my case, I suffered a massive stroke in 2006 and was placed in a medically induced coma for six days. In 1985 I had a seizure and my driver's license was revoked for six months. The doctor or hospital is responsible for notifying the D.M.V. when someone loses consciousness. In my case, for some unknown reason, I fell through the cracks and my driver's license was never suspended after my stroke in 2006.

While living as an inpatient at a rehab facility I was offered drivers training classes as part of my rehab. To qualify, as a condition to the driver training, I would need a current driver's license with no restrictions and it had to be in good standing. After losing my driver's license when I had the seizure and being aware of the law, I was concerned that my license would have been revoked after the stroke, and therefore I would not be eligible to participate in the driver's training program. Someone told me to call the D.M.V. to inquire about the current status of my driver's license. The next morning I called the department of motor vehicles in Sacramento and asked the young lady who handled my call "if there were any restrictions on my driver's license"?

In the event that you do not know the status of your driver's license at the time of your call, you do not want to come right out and tell them that you have lost consciousness from a medical reason if you have done so. They could at that time start an investigation on your past medical status and start the process to revoking your driver's license. Instead you might say something like: "I am so and so from California and I think I might have parking tickets on my record. Could you please check to see if there are any tickets or any other restrictions on my driver's license"?

When I contacted the D.M.V. I was informed by them that I had no restrictions on my driver's license. Apparently the hospital failed to contact them after my stroke. With no restrictions on my driver's license, I went ahead and enrolled in the driver training at my rehab facility.

The driving program was designed to take into account the physical limitations I had from the result of the stroke. I was tested beforehand to check the issues I had that would affect me being able to drive safely. I completed the in car training over the next four weeks with no serious problems, although I knew my driving skill wasn't the same as before my stroke.

I returned home after being released from where I was living at a rehab facility and slowly began to drive again. I had suffered some brain injury from the massive stroke I had back in 2006. To this day I suffer from a condition that left me blind in the lower left sides of both eyes known as "left neglect".

I had friends who owned a driving school at the time. I went out with one of the instructors four or five times to drive around the local neighborhoods before I planned to drive solo. After that I started driving around my neighborhood by myself for a week or two to see how I would do when driving by myself. I soon started driving the three mile round trip to my real estate office and back a few times a week.

The "left neglect" left me with little to no peripheral vision to my left side. I can see 20/20 straight ahead, but the brain does not recognize anything out of the vision cut on the left side. I drove to and from my work over the next month with no apparent problems. I even made a three hour trip to west Los Angeles to run an errand. The trip to Los Angeles was extremely stressful and fraught with lots of near misses and close calls on the way. The first leg of the trip took so long that I decided to take the freeway home. It's like speeding up when you're lost. I realize now how foolish I was in making that drive that day.

Some days later while driving to my office, on a quiet two lane highway just a few miles from my home, I rear ended three Korean kids. With the total loss of my peripheral vision, I did not notice that they had pulled in front of me and stopped for some unknown reason. I never even saw them until I ran into them; I never even hit the brakes. Had they been standing out behind the car changing a tire I would have killed them all. After this accident I felt fortunate that no one was killed or seriously injured, and I elected never to drive again.

Since the accident I have developed a network of drivers made up of family and friends. I rely on these wonderful people to help get me get to church, doctor's appointments, and any of a number of speaking engagements I now need to make.

If you experience any medical condition that leaves you with any loss of vision or depth perception, you must be checked out and have some sort of driver's training before you attempt to drive again.

There will come a time when you feel you want to or need to drive following your stroke. Please do not get behind the wheel of an automobile until you have gone through the proper channels to safely return to driving again after your stroke. The wrong decision could haunt you for the rest of your life—I was lucky but you may not be.

Driver aids that make post stroke driving safer:

1. Stick on "fish eye" mirrors. These are placed on both outside rear view mirrors and will expand your vision to the rear and sides.

2. Oversized rear view mirror. This fits over your standard rear view mirror and allows you to see to the rear

both right and left more completely.

3. Brody knob. This device is bolted to your steering wheel on the strong side of the steering wheel. It is a door knob size knob that allows the user to rotate the steering wheel 360 degrees easily and using only the strong hand. It is a must for one handed drivers. I highly recommend these three devises to increase ease and safety for the post stroke driver.

Furthermore, I recommend that when and if you start driving after your stroke, that you try to eliminate any "left hand" turns from your driving, except when turning at a signal light or at a four way stop.

Always plan your trip out carefully before setting out. Plan to make more than one stop when going out, make a list of required stops beforehand, and combine multiple errands; this will minimize the amount of time you will spend behind the wheel.

Before getting behind the wheel of an automobile ask family or close friends if they notice anything about you that would lead them to think you might be unsafe when driving. These people know you best and they most likely knew you before your stroke.

If you have any vision, hearing or other physical impairments, think seriously about getting evaluated and getting some driving instruction from a professional before getting behind the wheel of a 2,000 pound guided missile and taking the chance at killing yourself, or worse someone else. If God forbid, you do kill someone:

When you are not safe to drive and you injure someone in an automobile accident, you will have to live with it for the rest of your life. You can be sued by the injured parties for everything you own.

It is not uncommon for stroke survivors to want to drive an automobile after having a debilitating stroke. Getting around to the many doctors' appointments and other responsibilities that require transportation may add pressure on the survivor whether to drive or not to drive following a stroke.

Driver safety is even more important when getting behind the wheel after a stroke. Any brain injury resulting in the loss of vision or depth perception issues should be closely monitored and considered before driving after stroke. Brain injury may affect the way you do things and cause you to be unsafe or even unable to safely drive after a stroke.

Before attempting to drive again after your stroke consult your doctor and a professional driving instructor trained in working with handicapped drivers. Some stroke survivors do not want to accept the mental or physical limitations that may leave them unsafe to drive after they suffer a life changing stroke. Many times stroke survivors feel they are able to drive when they are really not. That was the case with me, and it was fortunate that I did not kill myself or others by being too stubborn and selfish to know when to stop driving.

Driving against doctor's orders may not only be dangerous to yourself and others but be illegal as well. Unsafe driving after a stroke can leave you open to being sued. If you have had your driver's license revoked following a stroke and injure or kill someone in an automobile accident, you could face felony charges and even jail time. Many states obligate doctors to notify the Department of Motor Vehicles when they advise someone not to drive due to limited driving skills either mentally, physically, or both. You could not only lose your money or home but your freedom as well.

Vision and driving after stroke:

Vision impairments following a severe stroke may affect as many as half of all stroke survivors. Vision is a learned process that derives meaning from what is seen by the brain through the eyes. This process is a complex learned set of skills.

Survivors with brain injury and vision related impairments are many times misdiagnosed at their initial evaluation. Hidden or neglected vision problems many at times cause delays in the survivor's rehabilitation. Good vision is important to keep the flow of information coming from the eyes to the brain for processing.

If you plan to drive, you must know:

* Where "straight ahead" is located in relation to you at any given time.

* Know how far away or how close things are in relation to you. (Depth perception).

* Knowing where you really are in space and time.

* If you suffer with "double vision"; are you able to correct it on your own?

* Can you look ahead to one particular spot? If not, this could be a sign of a balance issue that may cause you to be unsafe to drive.

Clear unrestricted vision and proper depth perception are just a few of the important factors to safely operating an automobile after a stroke.

Handicap parking placards.

Handicap parking placards are a must and easy to obtain. Have your attending doctor or rehab facility write you a prescription for a handicap parking placard. Take or mail the prescription to your local D.M.V office, and the placard will be mailed to you within three to six weeks and will be automatically renewed every two years in the month of May in most states. They expire in the month of June.

The fines for parking in a handicap parking spot and not displaying a placard can run as high as one thousand dollars. It's preferred to hang the placard from the inside rear view mirror, but i had had no problems putting it on the dashboard in plain view with the expiration date face up.

If you happen to forget to post your handicap placard and do get a parking ticket. Take the ticket and your placard to the police station where the ticket was issued. You will need to fill out a form explaining the reason you failed to display your placard, and usually you will be charged a small processing fee to resend the parking citation that you can mail in. Usually the processing is $25.

Chapter 6

Eating After a Stroke

It is common to have trouble swallowing, also called dysphasia, after a stroke. You may not be able to feel food on one or both sides of your mouth. You may have problems chewing or producing enough saliva; Or you may have other conditions that make eating difficult and increase your risk of choking.

Other things that may interfere with normal eating include:

* Problems seeing or judging where things are, especially on the side of your body affected by the stroke.

* Problems recognizing familiar objects or remembering how to do everyday things.

* Paralysis or weakness or trouble controlling movements (apraxia).

* Problems with smell, taste, or the sense of feeling.

* Depression, which can cause a loss of appetite and may require treatment.

If you have eating problems after a stroke, you will need a thorough evaluation by a speech therapist or another rehabilitation specialist. You may need special x-rays to see how you are swallowing. As you recover from a stroke, your rehabilitation team will monitor your progress. Swallowing and eating problems often improve over time, but some may last for the rest of your life. But there are many things you can do to make eating easier

Preventing another stroke and staying healthy can be achieved when you take appropriate steps to control your weight and blood pressure. Making healthy food choices is a major step in the right direction, and you can enhance the impact diet plays in your stroke risk by meeting with a registered dietitian. A dietitian can teach you how to prepare and plan meals and snacks to enhance your health.

Healthy Food Groups:

* Grains: whole grains are best.
* Vegetables: choose often, nutrient-rich dark green, orange, and yellow vegetables and remember to regularly eat dried beans and peas.
* Fruits: eat a variety of fresh, frozen, or dried fruits each day.
* Dairy: choose low-fat or fat-free dairy foods.
* Protein: choose low-fat or lean meats, poultry; and remember to vary your choices with more beans, peas, nuts, seeds, and fish. In terms of fats. Limit fat intake from butter, stick margarine, shortening, or lard.

Eat a variety of foods each day.

Because no single food can provide our bodies with all of the nutrients we need for good health, choose a variety of foods each day.

Eat a rainbow of colorful foods at each meal.

In order to reap the health-protective nutrients found in fruits and vegetables, it's important to choose a variety of colorful foods at each meal. Go for a rainbow approach, by choosing an array of fruits, vegetables and legumes — dark reds, oranges, vibrant yellows, deep greens, blues, and purples. By choosing a rainbow of color to your diet you'll be sure to take in a wide range of nutrients.

Research shows that the best way to reap the benefits of a healthy diet is to bump up your fruits and vegetables. So, in addition to steps 1 and 2, make sure you eat a minimum of 5 servings each day.

Choke danger.

The part Bell's palsy plays on eating

What is Bell's palsy?
Bell's palsy is a paralysis or weakness of the muscles on one side of your face. Damage to the facial nerve that controls muscles on one side of the face causes that side of your face to droop . The nerve damage may also affect your sense of taste and how you make tears and saliva. This condition comes on suddenly, often overnight, and usually gets better on its own within a few weeks.

What causes Bell's palsy?
1. In most cases of Bell's palsy, the nerve that controls muscles on one side of the face is damaged by inflammation.

Many health problems can cause weakness or paralysis of the face. If a specific reason cannot be found for the weakness, the condition is called Bell's palsy.

Symptoms of Bell's palsy include:

* Sudden weakness or paralysis on one side of your face that causes it to droop. This is the main symptom. It may make it hard for you to close your eye on that side of your face.

* Drooling.

* Eye problems, such as excessive tearing or a dry eye.

* Loss of ability to taste.

* Pain in or behind your ear.

* Numbness in the affected side of your face.

* Increased sensitivity to sound.

Your doctor may diagnose Bell's palsy by asking you questions, such as about how your symptoms developed. He or she will also give you a physical and neurological exam to check facial nerve function.

Most people who have Bell's palsy recover completely, without treatment, in 1 to 2 months this is especially true for people who can still partly move their facial muscles. But a small number of people may have permanent muscle weakness or other problems on the affected side of the face.

Developing your strategy for safe eating after stroke

1. First and probably the most important step.

Be sure to work with your doctor and qualified speech therapist to find out your limits and develop strategies and safeguards to eating after stroke.

Some things that have worked well for me are as follows.

1. Slow down.

2. Identify foods you have proven to be able to EAT.

3. Chew food well before swallowing.

4. If your mouth is full, do not attempt to put any more food in it.

5. Take small bites. Clear your mouth before each bite.

6. Take sips of a liquid during and after meals to help you clear you mouth and throat.

7. As a last resort spit out the food you cannot swallow. It's unsettling to guests at the table with you, but it's better to offend someone than to choke to death on a mouthful of food you cannot get down.

Take heart and have patience. This condition can improve with time and the help of a good speech therapist. Practice and experiment to find the best strategies that works best for you and your limitations and condition.

My stratagems for safe eating

It's important to test and experiment with soft foods first. Not until you have been able to at least swallow thickened liquids and soft chopped or mashed foods should you attempt to swallow solid food.

Start out trying foods like: tomato soup, chicken broth, and then you might try a soft vegetable soup. Remember fibrous raw vegetables can be hard to chew. Fresh vegetables and bread should be considered a choke risk in the early stages of retraining to eat.

Since getting enough food value is difficult when getting

back to an unrestricted diet try to choose foods with high calorie counts and good food values.

Try foods that have been proven to be good starter foods, both easy to eat and high in nutritional value.

Foods like, apple sauce, mashed potatoes and gravy, hot cereals like cream of wheat and cooked oats are a good choice. The daily bowl of ice cream or pudding can give you some variation in your diet to change things up a bit. Yogurt and cottage cheese are also very good for you and are a good transitional food source. Go ahead and take it slow, all foods are optional; you just need to identify what you can safely eat. If you have to eat the same thing for every meal every day, so be it.

At the early stages of your eating recovery it would most likely be prudent to stay away from bread, french fries, and raw vegetables. Stewed vegetables may be acceptable. Chew each and every bite thoroughly and swallow at least three times for each bite you take. Keep bites relatively small and only put food into your mouth after swallowing what you already have in your mouth.

It's common for stroke survivors to do what I call the stroke shovel. It's when you fill your mouth with food and before clearing what is in the mouth, even when food is spilling out of your mouth, you continue to try to put more food into your mouth.

This is not only a losing battle and unappetizing to people dining with you but can be very dangerous and result in a choke hazard. Try to resist this urge and get in the habit of clearing your mouth of food before trying to put more in it. I have found that if you will put the silverware down every few bites it helps to slow your roll.

In the early stages of learning to eat again the use of your tongue is VERY important. Watch others eat. You use your whole mouth to eat. You use your tongue, lips, cheeks, and throat.

Your tongue is important, in that it is the primary muscle

in your mouth used to move the food around. The smaller the bite the easier it will be to be able to use the tongue to maneuver the food back and forth between your molars and teeth. The molars are used to break down the food or macerate it until the food is safe to swallow. Your lips and cheeks also play a large part in this chewing and maceration process.

Remember that the goal to stroke recovery is "safety first". If you get yourself into trouble by taking too much food into your mouth and it cannot be safely swallowed, you can always spit it out into a napkin.

It's almost a given that in the early stages of retraining to eat again that one or more of these problems will occur multiple times. When dining, keep a stack of paper napkins on the table next to your plate.

It is better to spit out some food and take a chance of offending someone than to choke to death on something you cannot safely swallow.

As with the other retraining and recovery processes with patience and practice, eating will get easier and safer in time.

Aspiration pneumonia is bronchopneumonia that develops due to the entrance of foreign materials into the bronchial tree,[1] usually oral or gastric contents (including food, saliva, or nasal secretions). Depending on the acidity of the aspirate, a chemical pneumonitis can develop, and bacterial pathogens (particularly anaerobic bacteria) may add to the inflammation.

After a stroke you will be at an increased risk for developing pneumonia, your medical needs include making sure you do not get liquids or food particles into your lungs. Most survivors have had to be on thickened liquids to help reduce the chance of getting pneumonia.

Chapter 7

Getting Social Security, Disability and Medicare Started. Don't Wait!!

After your stroke, as soon as you are able present yourself to your nearest SSSi-Disability office. You can get the number from 411 information. Request a face to face appointment with an authorized officer at the office nearest to you. Explain your circumstances and ask for advice on how to proceed and what benefits you qualify for. Also request all forms needed to get started.

Remember, the sooner you get started the sooner your benefits will start. There is a waiting period before any claim is paid out. You may be eligible for disability, social security, and Medicare. These could be the difference of living comfortably or going broke.

If you can make the trip, you should try to go in person, if not a power of attorney can get the ball rolling for you. Them seeing you in person, and that you are in some ways handicapped after your stroke may help your case. I know it did in mine.

If you cannot make the appointment, send a caregiver with a power of attorney.

Time is of the essence, do not wait!!

Benefits for people with disabilities

The social security and supplemental security income disability programs are the largest of several federal programs that provide assistance to people with disabilities. While these two programs are different in many ways, both are administered by the social security administration, and only individuals who have a disability and meet medical criteria may qualify for benefits under either program.

Social security disability insurance pays benefits to you and certain members of your family if you are "insured," meaning that you worked long enough and paid social security taxes.

Supplemental security income pays benefits based on financial need.

When you apply for either program, we will collect medical and other information from you and make a decision about whether or not you meet social security's definition of disability.

Use the benefits eligibility screening tool to find out which programs may be able to pay you benefits.

If your application has recently been denied, the internet appeal is a starting point to request a review of our decision about your eligibility for disability benefits.

If your application is denied for:

* Medical reasons, you can complete and submit the required appeal request and appeal disability report online.

The disability report asks you for updated information about your medical condition and any treatment, tests or doctor visits since we made our decision.

* Non-medical reasons, you should contact your local social security office to request the review. You also may call our toll-free number, 1-800-772-1213, to request an appeal. People who are deaf or hard of hearing can call our toll-free tty number, 1-800-325-0778.

Applying for social security and disability insurance following your stroke.

First and foremost. You must gather all your papers from your doctors. You then get them all in order and make an appointment for as soon as possible with the social security office. They will set you up for an interview.

At this time bring all your paperwork to the department with you. After your interview it will take several weeks before you are contacted by them.

When you finally hear from them, do not be discouraged if you are turned down. This can happen some of the time when you first file.

They will give you a lot of paperwork, be sure you complete every page. If everything is not filled in and completed this will slow down an already slow process. They will try again to discourage you from filing for benefits. You must not give up and reapply again.

This will not happen overnight. But you must remember, you have worked your whole life and you are entitled to your hard earned benefits. It is not a gift; you have earned it by the many years you have paid into the fund.

Remember God is with you, he is your healer and strength and always with you in spirit.

If you experience a lot of grief from SSI&SDI, you may need to hire a lawyer, many folks end up needing one to get what is rightly theirs.

Chapter 8

Healing Through
Breathing and Meditation

The work that follows is meant to be only an abbreviated lesson on meditation. If you have a positive experience, I recommend you find further instruction. At the end of this lesson I will instruct you further in finding the next steps you will need to take for self-meditation.

Meditation has been used for hundreds of years in Asia to obtain many positive results. Healing, relaxing; and the elusive enlightenment" or the (meaning to life).

When preparing one's self for meditation, you will need to find a comfortable place to sit or lay. Wherever you decide to do your meditation try to do it in the same place each time. It is important to keep your back straight when meditating.

Make sure to be in a quiet place with no distractions. I have found it conducive to meditation to be in a warm environment with non-restrictive clothing.

The unique state of restful alertness gained during the transcendental meditation technique promotes health by reducing activation of the sympathetic nervous system — which, in turn, dilates the blood vessels and reduces stress hormones, such as adrenaline, noradrenalin. The importance of breathing in meditation — breathing for health.

Life is but a series of breaths. Breath is life. We can live a long time without food, a couple of days without drinking water, but life without breath is measured in seconds. Something so essential deserves our attention. Breath is the most important of all the bodily functions.

Proper breathing is one of the most important things you can do for maintaining your health. There is a right way and a wrong way to breathe. Children breathe deeply, from their diaphragm. As we age, however, our breathing shifts to the chest and becomes shallower and more rapid. Deep breathing is best.

I recommend taking a few minutes each day to practice breathing deeply. You'll find a breathing exercise at the end of this page to help you learn to breathe more deeply throughout the day.

Pranamaya: a simple breathing exercise you can use in your daily routine

Are you willing to invest just 5 minutes a day in a breathing exercise which will produce immediate and significant benefits? The ayurvedic breathing technique known as "pranayama" is a tremendously beneficial practice for your health and it's free.

Health through breathing by Danny Jones

What follows are some simple breathing exercises that have worked well for me. Also a short lesson on meditation follows the breathing segment. Both subjects can be found online; books and tapes can be purchased if you want further instruction. Start slow and see if you get any benefit from my instruction first. Enjoy.

The relaxing breath

Step 1: For this exercise we start by placing the tongue in the "yogic position". Start by touching the tip of your tongue to the back of your front teeth, and then slide it back to the hard ridge of the pallet. Lightly touch this ridge with the tip of your tongue. You will leave the tongue in this position throughout the exercise.

Step 2: Exhale completely through your mouth.

Step 3: Close your mouth and inhale through your nose for the count of four seconds and hold the breath for seven seconds.

Step 4: Now exhale through your mouth for a count of eight seconds.

The ratio of the inhale, hold and exhale is the important part, not how long it takes to do the exercise. As you practice the steps try to slow the steps down, remember to keep the 4, 7, 8 ratio.

This exercise works well if you get upset with something or someone, it will help to slow the mind and body and relives stress. It also is a very powerful sleep aid.

The refreshing breath

For this exercise, you will breathe in and out through the nose only, keep your mouth lightly closed for the duration of the exercise.

Step1: Start with the tongue in the "yogic" position, as described above (relaxing breath). Leave tongue in "yogic" position throughout the exercise.

Step2: Exhale completely through your mouth, close mouth.

Step3: Now breathe in and out through your nose rapidly. The goal is to get three breath cycles per second. Inhalation and exhalation should be of equal length.

Start by doing this rapid breath in and out of your nose for fifteen seconds at a time.

Do this exercise at least three times a day to start with. Every day you can add five seconds to the duration of the breath.

The goal is to work up to a full minute and a half of the rapid in and out, three breath cycles per second through the nose only.

The use of this breath is an excellent way to dissipate fatigue/stress. It also works well to wake yourself up. If you become sleepy, just do the exercise a few minutes and you will find it is a great way to wake yourself up.

Being at one with the universe

This breath takes some active imagination. I imagine the

"Holy Spirit" in the place of the universe, it works well for me.

Step 1. Start by lying flat on your back with arms comfortably by your side. Breathe in and out for one minute. Breathe out for 3 second Count, in for 3 sec. Count.

Continue breathing in, out, now imagine the universe spread out above you.

Step 2. Now pretend that you are not doing the breathing but the universe is breathing for you.

When you exhale it is like the universe is withdrawing the breath from your lungs. And when you inhale the universe is blowing breath into you.

Remember you are not doing the breathing, the universe is breathing you. Now imagine yourself floating in the air above you in space. Continue to breathe in and out… the universe is breathing completely for you as you float gently in space.

Now picture yourself as a tiny but important part of the universe.

Step 3: If you can, remember that throughout this exercise to keep breath cycles at 2-3 seconds in, out.

This is an excellent sleep aid. You can do this exercise to help you go to sleep or when just waking up in the morning. It will give a calming effect for several hours after doing the exercise.

Combing the relaxing breath and the refreshing breaths

Try combining the two breaths. Start with doing the relaxing breath first followed with the refreshing breath next, in and out through the nose three times a second for one minute.

You will find that that is a great way to start your meditation.

The goal in your breathing is that it needs to be deeper, quieter, slower and more regular.

Start by breathing in then out regularly for a minute or more, then make a concentrated effort to make your breathing deeper, quieter, slower, and more regular.

This is the goal: try doing this for three times a day for the first month, then increase the process by another minute till you get up to five minutes three times a day.

This will help regulate your respiration, stabilize your heart rate, and slow your blood pressure down. Your body will relax and your mind will become peaceful.

Squeezing more air out of the lungs:

The more air you can move through your lungs the better.

Start by breathing in and out regularly. Now exhale out of your mouth completely. When you get to the end, squeeze out a little more air, and then a little more. If you can, when exhaling, at the end of every breath squeeze a little more air out of your lungs.

It makes sense that the more air you can exhale, the more air you are to inhale.

The 3&3 breath

Practice this breath just before you start mediation. I call it the 3&3 breath. When you are relaxed and tension free, try the 3&3 breath.

Start out by breathing regularly in and out; try not to influence your breath in any way. Do this for a minute or two.

Inhale through your nose for a count of three seconds, hold for three seconds. Now exhale through your mouth for a count of three seconds. Do this sequence for three to five minutes. I have found this breath to be a good sleep aid. Try it when preparing to fall asleep.

I have found that combining several breathing exercises can help to intensify the meditation experience.

With practice and some experimentation you will find

what works best for you.

Meditation—the key to less stress and more rest and relaxation.

We cannot eliminate the stress in our day to day lives, but we can learn how to manage the stress we do have, better.

Step 1: Sit or lie with your back kept straight. It's important for your breathing that your spine is straight. Make sure you are in a warm quiet place. Make sure that your clothing is loose fitting and does not bind you. You can leave your eyes closed, open, or half open.

When you are comfortable and breathing regularly, say to yourself "I am releasing all the stress and tension from my mind and body". Repeat this to yourself three times.

Then say: "I am releasing all the tension in my feet and ankles". Then say: I am releasing all the tension in my calf and thigh muscles.

Then say: "I am releasing all the tension in my belly and lower back".

Then say: "I am releasing the tension in my chest, shoulders, and back muscles".

Then release the tension in your arms and hands.

Lastly release the tension in your neck, face, and scalp.

Now tell yourself: "My mind is becoming calm and peaceful".

Now tell yourself: "I am now focusing on my body".

Tell yourself: "My heart rate and breathing are steady and unrestrained. I am now free of all stress and tension in my body and mind".

"I am relaxed and my mind is fully at peace". (Repeat saying this to yourself 3 times)

In this relaxed state you will continue breathing in a regular steady manner. In and out in and out. Do this for a few minutes, in and out in and out. Inhale deeply through your nose and exhale completely through your mouth.

Now just follow your breath, in and out...

Tell yourself: My mind and body are one".

Tell yourself: "I am now fully in the present". "I am comfortable and completely at peace with myself and the world around me".

Feel your breath expanding your lungs. Notice where you feel the breath. Is it through the nose; is it the air through the mouth expanding your lungs?

It doesn't matter where you feel your breath, just be aware of where you observe it. Concentrate on each breath.

Breath is the most natural object of meditation. Now just follow the breath, in and out, in and out... as you concentrate on your breath, thoughts and concerns may enter your mind. When they do just return to following the breath, in and out, in and out, just follow the breath. Whenever unwanted thoughts enter your mind, gently return to following the breath, in and out, in and out.

Now tell yourself: "I am completely relaxed and deeply in a state of meditation. I am fully in the moment and will not let the cares of the world upset me".

When you feel you are done meditating, tell yourself: "I am at one with my mind and body. When I awake I will be at peace with the world. I will awake relaxed and stress free".

You can repeat these steps as many times as you wish. Learn to use breath work and meditation to achieve a sense of wellbeing.

You can do this in any quiet place; it requires no equipment, is drug free, and does not cost you any money.

Most of the things we worry about do not ever happen, and the ones that do happen are usually not as bad as we expected. Your worrying will never change the outcome.

Good rule for breathing and meditation:

Start with twenty minutes of breathing exercises. Then spend ten minutes de stressing and relaxing your mind and body. Then spend twenty minutes in meditation. It helped me to dedicate a time each day to doing my breathing work.

Chapter 9

My Stroke July 21st 2006

My warning signs were cold sweats, soaking sweats, and shakes.

I Thought I had overworked or had a relapse from working on my rental house. I woke up and was unable to get myself off the floor. I was also unable to raise by left arm.

Endocarditis:

Endocarditis is an infection of the inner lining of your heart.

The disease typically occurs when bacteria or other germs from another part of your body, such as your mouth, spread through your bloodstream and attach to damaged areas in your heart. Left untreated, Endocarditis can damage or destroy your heart valves and can lead to life-threatening complications. Treatments for Endocarditis include antibiotics and, in severe cases, surgery.

Endocarditis is uncommon in people with healthy hearts. People at greatest risk of Endocarditis have a damaged heart valve or an artificial heart valve.

Causes, incidence, and risk factors

Endocarditis can involve the heart muscle, heart valves, or lining of the heart. Most people who develop Endocarditis have had some abnormality of a heart valve.

Risk factors for developing Endocarditis include:

Injection drug use

Permanent central venous access lines

Prior valve surgery

Recent dental surgery

Weakened valves

Bacterial infection is the most common source of Endocarditis.

The orthopedic group that preformed my spinal fusion neither tested me or asked me if i had a condition called Mitro prolapse. And i did. This condition is thought to be what caused the Endocarditis which ultimately caused the stroke I suffered in July of 2006

Heart murmurs: heart murmurs are abnormal sounds during your heartbeat cycle — such as whooshing or swishing — made by turbulent blood in or near your heart. These sounds can be heard with a stethoscope. A normal heartbeat makes two sounds like "lubb-dupp" (sometimes described as "lub-dup"), which are the sounds of your heart valves opening and closing.

Heart murmurs can be present at birth (congenital) or develop later in life. A heart murmur isn't a disease — but murmurs may indicate an underlying heart problem.

Most heart murmurs are harmless (innocent) and don't require treatment. Some heart murmurs may require follow-up tests to be sure the murmur isn't caused by a serious underlying heart condition. Treatment, if needed, is directed at the cause of your heart murmur.

Mitro prolapse

Mitral valve prolapse symptoms

What are the symptoms and signs of mitral valve prolapse?

Most people with mitral valve prolapse have no symptoms, however, those who do, commonly complain of symptoms such as fatigue, palpitations, chest pain, anxiety, and migraine headaches. Stroke is a very rare complication of mitral valve prolapse.

What is mitral valve prolapse?

In patients with mitral valve prolapse, the mitral apparatus (valve leaflets and chordae) becomes affected by a process called myxomatous degeneration. In myxomatous degeneration, the structural protein collagen forms abnormally and causes thickening, enlargement, and redundancy of the leaflets and chordae. When the ventricles contract, the redundant leaflets prolapse (flop backwards) into the left atrium, sometimes allowing leakage of blood through the valve opening (mitral regurgitation). When severe, mitral regurgitation can lead to heart failure and abnormal heart rhythms. Most patients are totally unaware of the prolapsing of the mitral valv.

Hemiplegia

Classification and external resources
Hemiplegia /he.mə .pliː .dʒ iə / is total paralysis of the arm, leg, and trunk on the same side of the body. Hemiplegia is more severe than hemiparesis, wherein one half of the body has less marked weakness.[1] hemiplegia may be congenital or acquired from an illness or stroke.

Hemiplegia is not an uncommon medical disorder. In elderly individuals, strokes are the most common cause of hemiplegia. In children, the majority of cases of hemiplegia has no identifiable cause and occurs with a frequency of about one in every thousand births. Experts indicate that the majority of cases of hemiplegia that occur up to the age of two should be considered to be cerebral palsy until proven otherwise.

Left neglect.

Hemispatial neglect is most frequently associated with left neglect.

Hemispatial neglect results most commonly from brain injury to the right cerebral hemisphere, causing visual neglect of the left-hand side of space. Right-sided spatial neglect is rare because there is redundant processing of the right space by both the left and right cerebral hemispheres, whereas in most left-dominant brains the left space is only processed by the right cerebral hemisphere. Although most strikingly affecting visual perception ('visual neglect'), neglect in other forms of perception can also be found, either alone, or in combination with visual neglect.

For example, a stroke affecting the right parietal lobe of the brain can lead to neglect for the left side of the visual field, causing a patient with neglect to behave as if the left side of sensory space is nonexistent. In an extreme case, a patient with neglect might fail to eat the food on the left half of their plate, even though they complain of being hungry. If someone with neglect is asked to draw a clock, their drawing might show only numbers 12 to 6, or all 12 numbers on one half of the clock face, the other side being distorted or left blank. Neglect patients may also ignore the affected side of their body, shaving, or adding make-up only to the non-neglected side. These patients may frequently collide with objects or structures such as door frames on the side being neglected.

Neglect may also present as a delusional form, where the patient denies ownership of a limb or an entire side of the body.

Neglect not only affects present sensation but memory and recall perception as well. A patient suffering from neglect may also, when asked to recall a memory of a certain object and then draw said object, again, only draw half of the object.

I had to be catheterized every four hours 24/7 the first six months following my stroke. My urinary specialist chose to not put the more permanent leg bag with a stay-in catheter in me. He thought that that would make my bladder lazy and increase the chance of it never coming back in.

Ischemic stroke occurs when a blood vessel that supplies blood to the brain is blocked by a blood clot. This may happen in two ways:

* A clot may form in an artery that is already very narrow. This is called a thrombotic stroke.

* A clot may break off from another place in the blood vessels of the brain, or from some other part of the body, and

travel up to the brain. This is called cerebral embolism, or an embolic stroke.

Ischemic strokes may be caused by clogged arteries. Fat, cholesterol, and other substances collect on the artery walls, forming a sticky substance called plaque. There are two major types of stroke: ischemic stroke and hemorrhagic stroke.

The cause of my stroke on 4/20/2006: I was broadsided by a car that ran a red light resulting in a neck injury to my neck and totaling my car.

On 5/31/06 I started treatment for my neck injury. I went to a local orthopedic group for diagnosis and treatment for my injury on 5/31/06. I was given pain medication and scheduled for P.T and an MRI. On 6/3/2005. When the MRI was read it showed I had ruptured discs at c-6 and c-7. I was then scheduled for surgery. First at St. Jude, then I was changed to Fullerton surgery center where they did my spinal fusion as an outpatient On 1/31/06 with a doctor who worked with the orthopedic group. My wife and I informed them that our insurance would not cover the procedure at an outpatient center, but they proceeded anyway. They were having difficulty with me in the recovery room but released me anyway after five hours. It was terrible. I was just about kicked out the door after major surgery. I now realize that I should have listened to my brother-in-law, Jim Goatcher, and had received a second opinion from a neurologist. I got home, and that night had to swallow medications. They did the surgery through my mouth. And five hours later I was home in my bedroom. I almost strangled to death from the lack of a suction devise to clear the saliva.

Three to four months following surgery, I started experiencing severe night sweats, chills, and low grade fever with moderate to severe low back pain. I was prescribed more pain medication.

Two days before my stroke on 7/17/06 I was seen by a doctor at the orthopedic group. While in front of him, I had an episode of sweats and racking chills. He did nothing and prescribed more pain medication. He did not offer any advice and I was not told to consult my primary doctor.

On 7/21/06 I was rushed by ambulance to St. Jude hospital. Where following tests. A cat scan, EKG, EEG, and others. It was determined that I had suffered a massive stroke to the right side of my brain caused by the blood disease Endocarditis.

The blockage was caused by the vegetative state of my mitro valve. The infectious control Doctor at St. Jude hospital ran tests and stated it was a staph Infection. My cardiologist Doctor at St. Jude explained to my wife that I had had mitral prolapse and the deformed leaflets will attract and harbor any blood infection. It was explained to me that my Mitro valve, the heart valve in the left side of your heart, has "leaflets" that look similar the tentacles on a sea anemone. When the Endocarditis attacks the heart valve, the name for the damage that occurs is "vegetative state". I was told that my heart was damaged severely at that time. And one day in the future I would need open heart surgery to replace the damaged heart valve with a new mechanical heart valve.

I had had no dental work or any other medical procedures other than the spinal fusion. There was no other source that I could have contracted the Endocarditis. The infectious doctor put me through a six week course of intravenous antibiotics to kill the infection.

On 9/5/06 I was deemed to be infection free and was soon transferred to Casa Colina in Pomona California. I was going to be living at the "TLC" unit or the "transitional care" unit. It was located on the hospital property.

My back continued to hurt and got increasingly painful. I was unable to get through the sessions with my occupational therapy and especially physical therapy. This was relayed to my rehab doctor. He did an emergency MRI. When that had be done and read, I was sent by ambulance to valley community hospital a few miles away from Casa Colina on 9/25/06. Where I was quickly admitted and tests were ordered. The doctor ordered blood tests and a lumbar disc biopsy. They found I had a staph infection of the disc in my spine. I was treated with strong antibiotics once again. They thought I got the Staph infection when I had received several blood infusions at St. Jude hospital when being treated for anemia. Doctor Daniel Gluckstien the director of infectious diseases at Casa Colina told me he thought that the staff infection could have only come from the spinal fusion. He thought there was no other way for it to have been introduced into my system, since blood is cleaned and sterilized.

Heart murmurs unsafe at any age, and what is a heart murmur?

A heart murmur is an extra or unusual sound heard during a heartbeat. Murmurs range from very faint to very loud. Sometimes they sound like a whooshing or swishing noise.

Normal heartbeats make a "lub-dupp" or "lub-dub" sound. This is the sound of the heart valves closing as blood moves through the heart. Doctors can hear these sounds and heart murmurs using a stethoscope.

The two types of heart murmurs are innocent (harmless) and abnormal.

Innocent heart murmurs aren't caused by heart problems. These murmurs are common in healthy children. Many children will have heart murmurs heard by their doctors at some point in their lives.

In adults, abnormal heart murmurs most often are caused by acquired heart valve disease. This is heart valve disease that develops as the result of another condition. Infections, diseases, and aging can all cause heart valve disease in otherwise healthy adults.

A heart murmur isn't a disease, and most murmurs are harmless. Innocent murmurs don't cause symptoms. Having one doesn't require you to limit your physical activity or do anything else special. Although you may have an innocent murmur throughout your life, you won't need treatment for it.

Treating muscle spasticity:

One in five stroke survivors suffer from painful muscle spasms. That result when weakened muscles contract abnormally. Someone with muscle spasticity may have a tight fist, an abnormally bent arm, a stiff knee, or a pointed foot. Not only are these spasms extremely painful but they can interfere with walking or performing routine tasks. Left untreated, muscle spasticity may deform a stroke survivor's limbs, restrict his ability to move, and lead to pressure sores.

Treatment for muscle spasticity may be a mix of rehabilitation therapies, medications, and even surgery if severe.

*Therapies may include full range-of-motion exercises several times a day, gentle stretching of tight muscles, and frequent repositioning of body parts.

*Oral medications include tizanidine, baclofen, benzodiazepines (like valium and klonopin), and dantrolene sodium.

*Injected medications include botulinum toxin (also known as botox), which targets specific muscles and lasts for up to three months. Injected phenol can alleviate pain for up to three years.

*Surgery can block pain and restore some movement. But because of potential complications, it's usually a last resort.

As the caregiver of someone with muscle spasticity, you can help him manage it and get the right treatments.

*Keep an eye out for "frozen" joints. If they are having trouble moving their arm or leg, try bending it for them. If it feels unusually stiff, that's most likely due to muscle spasm.

*Keep track of when and where spasms occur. Also ask their nurses and rehabilitation team what positions typically set off muscle spasms.

Paralysis and spasticity

Paralysis is the inability of a muscle or group of muscles to move voluntarily. When messages from the brain to the muscles won't work properly due to a stroke, a limb becomes paralyzed or develops a condition called spasticity.

Spasticity is tight, stiff muscles that make movement, especially of the arms or legs, difficult or uncontrollable. This condition can include any of the following: a tight fist, bent elbow, arm pressed against the chest, stiff knee and/or pointed foot that can interfere with walking. The spasms produce a pain similar to muscle cramping.

My experience with spasms
Subluxation
Shoulder subluxation
What is a shoulder subluxation?

A shoulder subluxation is a temporary, partial dislocation of the shoulder joint. The shoulder is a ball and socket joint. The ball of the upper arm bone (humorous) is held into the socket of the shoulder blade (scapula) by a group of ligaments.

How does it occur?

A shoulder subluxation can occur from falls onto your outstretched arm, direct blows to your shoulder, or having your arm forced into an awkward position. If you have had a previous injury or if your shoulder ligaments are naturally loose you may sublux your shoulder doing simple activities like throwing or putting on a shirt or jacket.

What are the symptoms?

Symptoms of a shoulder subluxation include:

* The feeling that your shoulder is going "in and out of joint"

* Looseness in your shoulder

* Pain, weakness, or numbness in your shoulder or arm

Your doctor will talk to you about your symptoms and perform a physical exam. Many times the diagnosis of a shoulder subluxation is made by your description of the injury. When your doctor examines you they may find that your shoulder is loose and may partially slip out of joint during the exam. Your doctor may order x-rays to see if you have had any fractures.

The pain from a shoulder subluxation is treated with ice packs for 20 to 30 minutes, 2 to 3 times a day. You may take an anti-inflammatory medication if prescribed by your attending doctor, like ibuprofen. You may need to avoid painful activities until the pain subsides.

The most important treatment for the looseness in the shoulder that causes a subluxation is shoulder strengthening exercises. Shoulders that continue to sublux and cause pain and cause painful symptoms may require surgery to correct the joint looseness.

The goal of rehabilitation is to return you to your sport or activity as soon as is safely possible. If you return too soon, you may worsen your injury; which could lead to permanent damage. Take your time to heal properly from an injury, or subluxation caused from stroke or other medical condition.

My Fall

My fall:
On 7/09/12 while going from the couch to the coffee pot in our kitchen at home, I had made the trip a thousand times since returning home after my stroke. I lost my balance and when I started to fall over, I was unable to stop myself from falling.

I fell to my weak side and landed with the full weight of my body on my left hand and wrist. Before I knew it, I had severely fractured my left hand and wrist. Like old men do that are too stubborn to go to the doctor or call 911 when they have chest pain and then die from a stroke or heart attack, I also refused to go to the hospital and get checked out after my fall.

I started self-medicating myself with pain killers I had on

hand. I foolishly thought that if I waited a few days it would quit hurting and just go away. After all it was my paralyzed arm; I could not use it anyway.

Unfortunately that can be a common way of thinking for stroke survivors. But nothing is further from the truth. Many serious conditions may develop from untreated injuries. It's better to error on the side of caution. You not only put your overall health at risk but put undue concern and worry on those who care for you.

If you take a fall and think you have injured yourself? Do not wait! Tell a caregiver, spouse, or call 911 immediately. Especially if you have struck your head in a fall. You may not experience pain after a fall but could have underlying injuries that could become life threatening. Bleeding to the brain does not always cause significant pain, and can end up being fatal if gone untreated. "NEVER", and I stress never, walk without a walking aid, (cane or walker) or get out of your wheelchair on your own unless you have doctor's orders to do so.

I waited a full week to go to the doctors following my fall. I was informed by the attending orthopedic doctor that if I had missed the ten day cutoff period for setting my hand and wrist that it may have healed crooked and I would most likely had to have had surgery to ever have them heal correctly.

A common misconception of stroke survivors is that "if I hurt myself on one of my "weak" or paralyzed limbs it does not matter, I cannot use them anyway". If you think you have been injured by a fall, there is a very good chance you have been. ONCE AGAIN, after a fall make sure to be checked out carefully.

Chapter 10

Positive Visualization
and Reconnection Exercises

Brain to muscle reconnection:
Milton Hyland Erickson TOLD BY DR. GOLAY 7/23/12
The following story was told to me by my psychologist Dr. Keith Golay during a session we had. We were discussing a subject I was working at called, Positive Visualization. He proceeded to tell me the true story of the work done by this amazing man.

This story is proof that positive visualization can work in some cases and does have medical merit. It might well be worth trying out, you have only your time to lose.

Milton Erickson was born on a farm in Lowell, Wisconsin. When a teenager at the age of seventeen he was stricken with polio. He soon lost all function in his limbs and could only move his eyes. He and his family would communicate by the blinking of the eyes.

He was totally bedridden at this time. Every day when the family would have to leave to work on the farm they would put Milton in an old rocking chair and move him in front of a window.

His mother, who was his main caregiver, would place him in a rocking chair with a hole cut in the seat because he had lost control of his bowels. She would then tie him safely into the rocker and push him over to the window where he could look out over the farmland. This came to be his only escape from the dreadful disease we know as polio. This became his daily routine most every day.

One morning his mother was called away unexpectedly and forgot to move him to his position in front of the window. He was secured in the rocking chair but was some distance from the window he longed to look out of.

He soon started imagining what he would be seeing if he was at "his spot" in front of the window looking out over the farm. He considered it his job to look out over the farm and see what was going on.

All of a sudden, as he was sitting there wishing he could see out the window located across the room, he was aware of a slight movement in his body. He was not sure what or where the movement came from.

Being a very observant person for most of his life, he started practicing and imagining being over by the window. He found that if he would imagine moving a particular muscle there was the slightest response to the thought he gave to that muscle.

Noticing the thought-response, he decided to start working on the movement process daily.

This would be the birth of "positive" visualization as we know it.

He would start working this new process on his hand and fingers, mostly because he could readily see them from where he sat. For the next several months he would work on the movement in his hand and fingers every day.

He started by thinking and imagining moving his index finger, after a few weeks he could move his index finger very slightly just a "twitch" at first. He would move to the next finger and repeat the process.

Over the next years he was able to "reactivate more and more muscle groups in his paralyzed body. Over a number of years Milton Erickson was able to rehabilitate his entire body from the ravages of polio.

He was the first person on record to actually be able to to do this—rehabilitate oneself with "Positive visualization". He was also the father of modern "hypnosis". He did early work to help with developing techniques for occupational therapy.

Milton Erickson eventually became a physician and completely restored himself from the effects of polio, and became a "post" polio patient.

If he could do it, why can't you? Give it a try and see what comes out of it.

Born 5 December 1901

Aurum, Nevada

Erickson frequently drew upon his own experiences to provide examples of the power of the unconscious mind. He was largely self-taught and a great many of his anecdotal and autobiographical teaching stories are collected by Sidney Rosen in the book My Voice Will Go With You. Erickson identified many of even his earliest personal experiences as hypnotic or auto hypnotic.

He grew up in Lowell, Wisconsin, in a farming family and intended to become a farmer like his father.

At age 17, he contracted polio and was so severely paralyzed that the doctors believed he would die.

Recovering, still almost entirely lame in bed, and unable to speak, he became strongly aware of the significance of non-verbal communication body language, tone of voice, and the way that these non-verbal expressions often directly contradicted the verbal ones.

He had polio, and was totally paralyzed, and the inflammation was so great that he had sensory paralysis too. Erickson could move his eyes, and his hearing was undisturbed. He got very lonesome lying in bed, unable to move anything except his eyeballs. He was quarantined on the farm with seven sisters, one brother, two parents, and a practical nurse. And how could he entertain himself? He started watching people.

He began to recall "body memories" of the muscular activity of his own body. By concentrating on these memories, he slowly began to regain control of parts of his body to the point where he was eventually again able to talk and use his arms. Still unable to walk, he decided to train his body further, by embarking—alone—on a thousand mile canoe trip with only a few dollars. After this grueling trip, he was able to walk with a cane. This experience may have contributed to Erickson becoming independent for the first time.

My work with positive visualization over one year: BY DANNY JONES

Step1. Start by lying on your back with your arms by your side. The prone position seems to work best for this work. It is work so rest when you feel you need to. Like we did with mediation, we start positive visualization by releasing the stress and tension in our bodies. Start by telling yourself:

"I am now releasing the tension in my body. I am releasing the tension in my feet, ankles, and legs. I am releasing the tension in my chest and back. I am releasing the tension in my shoulders, arms, and hands. I am releasing the tension in my face, neck, and head.

Now tell yourself I am completely free of stress and tension in my mind and body.

Step 2. Start by concentrating on your weak side leg, ankle, and foot.

Tell yourself: "I am now connecting my ankle through the Nero pathways of my left foot to my brain.

Tell yourself I am pressing my foot downward, now upward. I am bending my ankle up now down. Visualize the ankle movement in your mind. Up down up down. Do this movement for 3 sets of ten or for thirty repetitions. At the beginning of each set tell yourself "I am now connecting my ankle through the neuro pathways to my brain.

Now visualize wiggling your toes. Concentrate making the connection from the brain to your toes and spend five minutes on this step.

Now tell yourself: "I am now connecting my foot through the neuro pathways to my brain". Now see yourself in your mind's eye, moving your foot up then down, and side to side. Try not to move your leg, only the foot. Do this movement 30 times, side to side, up and down.

Step 3. Tell yourself: "I am now connecting my arm through the neuro pathways in my arm to my brain. "I am going to be able to raise my arm up off the bed. Visualize yourself raising your arm up and over your head. See yourself make the movement. Do this for 3 sets of 10 or for 30 repetitions.

Tell yourself at the beginning of each set: "I am now connecting my arm to my brain", and work hard to find the connection. Search through your brain to find the connection. It's in there; you just have to find it.

"I'm raising my arm up, I'm letting it down, I'm raising my arm up, and I'm letting it down. Visualize the movement.

Now tell yourself: "I am now moving my arm inward, now I'm moving my arm outward. Inward, outward. Do this movement 3 sets of 10 or 30 times.

Step 4. We will now concentrate on our hand and fingers on our weak side.

Tell yourself: "I am now connecting my hand and fingers through the neuro pathways from my hand to my brain.

Starting with the little finger, visualize you being able to raise it up then down, up then down. Now move your little finger from side to side.

Repeat these steps for each finger, repeat the exercise for each finger twenty times.

Visualize each movement in your mind's eye. Start each finger with these words: "I am now connecting my finger to my brain; I am now moving my finger".

Visualize moving your fingers, up then down, up then down, and side to side.

Perform this movement for each finger 30 times.

Step 5. The wrist. Getting movement back to the wrist is "paramount" for getting "return" (or functional use) back to the hand and fingers.

Tell yourself: "I am now connecting my wrist through the neuro pathways in my arm to my brain".

Tell yourself: "I am now going to bend my wrist up, then down. I am now moving my wrist from side to side. Up, down, side to side.

Now concentrate on making the connection from your

brain to your wrist. You must search your brain for the connection. Visualize yourself making the connection and making the movement in your "mind's eye". Tell yourself: "I'm bending my wrist up, I'm bending my wrist down".

Do this wrist exercise for three sets of ten or thirty repetitions.

Step 6 the arm:

Start by telling yourself: "I am now pulling my arm back". In a motion similar to that of drawing a pistol from a holster, visualize pulling your arm back, now see yourself pushing your arm forward. Back, now forward; visualize each movement in your mind. As you see the motions exert the effort to make the movement.

Do this "drawing the pistol" exercise for 3 sets of 10 or 30 reps. At the beginning of each set tell yourself: "I am now connecting my arm through the neuro pathways in my arm to my brain.

It is very important that you "search" your brain for the connection to the muscle group you are looking to get "return"/movement to. The connection is hidden in there in your brain; work on finding the "pathways" you are looking for.

The key is telling yourself what movement you want to do and believing that you can make it. Also work to see yourself making the movements as you exert the effort to make the movements.

There is a school of thought that says if you can see it, you can do it, and good luck.

Practice these steps "daily". The amount of reps you perform is not as important as to you being consistent in doing the steps daily. If you can do the exercises twice a day, you should see some improvement in your range of motion in a few months.

Chapter 11

Am I Ready to Come Home

After your stroke you probably spent some time in a hospital, and if you have good insurance, hopefully you got to spend time in a good rehab facility.

When you have recovered and are able to travel and take some of your care on, you will hopefully get to return home, or at least to an assisted care facility.

Before making the trip home it is important to stress the need to have someone qualified to do a pre-returning home inspection. This inspection is usually a mandatory condition for release from most rehab facilities.

My home inspection was conducted by my occupational therapist before I was discharged from the rehab facility I was living at as an inpatient. The reason for this inspection is for the most part to insure your safety when returning to a home environment. The person conducting the inspection will look for the following:

Any obvious trip hazards, like rugs, higher than normal door thresholds, a safe place to bathe or shower, a safe place to sleep and eat, and to see if you can access any steps or stairs in the home. There may be more, but this gives you an idea of what they will be looking for.

If you have not returned home, I have included some of the things that you will need to get in order before you are able to be ready to return home to this important milestone of your stroke recovery.

1. You will need to be fall proof in either your walking, scooter, or wheel chair.

2. If you returned home in a wheel chair, it will be helpful to be able to safely transfer from the wheelchair to a chair, couch, toilet, or bed.

3. If needed, to be able to assist caregivers in your daily

care. Both in dressing and some of your required personal care.

4. To be able to feed yourself safely.

5. Have the ability to transfer in and out of a car safely if needed.

6. The ability to get to and use the toilet safely.

7. Have easy access to and be able to use a telephone. This is especially important in case you need to call for emergency services.

8. Have in place aids needed, like toilet extensions, shower bench, and personal care aids, like a body brush and wash.

9. Have in place any ramps needed to access your home when entering or exiting.

10. Any modifications needed to bathrooms, shower, or stairs as required for your safety.

11. Any modifications made to stairs and steps.

12. Will you be independent enough to be left alone for an extended period of time?

13. Are you able to manage your medications on a daily basis by yourself?

14. Do you have a place to do your daily care and dressing?

15. Do you need an electric shaver? Many men take blood thinners, and shaving with a blade shaver, even a safety razor, may put you at risk for cutting yourself. I used to shave in the shower but found that when I nicked myself shaving, the cut would not stop due to the blood thinners I was taking; I went to an electric shaver, problem solved.

If you have a full or part time caregiver or will be living in a care facility. Being able to assist in your care will help in your recovery. This is important to help foster increased independence and self-esteem which leads to increased self-worth.

A trained occupational therapist doing an inspection on your home or living area in a care facility can give you important information to what is required to insure you are safe and comfortable in your new living environment.

If you plan to live on the first floor of a two story home, make sure you have:

1. Access to a toilet, shower, or bathtub.

2. A bed that you can access easily and safely.

3. A safe uncluttered space to spend time in a living room, easy chair in front of a TV. or a computer space.

4. A designated place to eat your meals.

5. Access to a telephone.

6. Do you need added safety rails for stairs and steps in the home?

If you have answered no to any of the previous questions you will need to contact a professional as needed to help you work on the areas you will need to be safe enough to return home.

I will list again the steps you should be safe in. What, who AND HOW to see to get them accomplished.

Fall Prevention

Contact a physical therapist to help you in getting treatment and training for preventing falls and becoming fall safe when walking or moving around your living space.

Falls are common after stroke. If you are independent from the use of the wheelchair and if you are now ambulatory, you will need to be safe when walking with a cane or walker. You may ALREADY be independent of walking aids.

First and foremost, and maybe the most important issue you will face is to be completely fall-safe in your home. Falls in the home injure 2.5 million Americans every year in this country. Falls are the number one cause for hospitalization for persons who have suffered a stroke and responsible for 500,000 deaths nationwide every year.

Until you are released by a qualified psychical therapist you will not be safe enough to walk on your own, and if you have been instructed to use a cane or walker you must be sure to use them.

A common mistake made by stroke survivors is that they choose to walk without a walking aid when they are not safe enough to do so, like I did. I fell and severely fractured my hand and wrist when walking without my cane in my home. I know that some of us gauge our recovery by being able to walk unassisted. Take it slowly and keep safety first.

I developed the bad habit of not using my cane in the house because I could hang on to the furniture and walls to get around. Carrying my coffee cup and using my cane did not work well without spilling coffee. I even tried walking for a while in our neighborhood park without my cane. That morning making the trip from the kitchen to the couch, a trip I had made a thousand times. I stood up from the couch and took two steps toward the kitchen. Then it happened, when I started to fall over and I lost my balance I fell on my paralyzed arm and hand, breaking my hand and wrist in five places.

I mistakenly thought that if I just tried hard enough to walk without my cane, someday I would be able to do it. Wrong, my brain injury is the deciding factor, and most likely my balance will never return enough for me to walk independently from a cane.

Sheer will and determination is not enough to overcome "brain injury".

I think most survivors come to a place in our recovery where we think we are ready to walk independent of a walking aid. But once again, your psychical therapist must sign off before you can walk without an aid.

Every year, one in every three adults age 65 and older will fall. Falls can cause moderate to severe injuries such as hip fractures, breaking of a limb, and head traumas, and can increase the risk of early death. Fortunately, falls are a public health problem that is largely preventable.

* Falls are the most common cause of traumatic brain injuries (TBI) in 2000, TBI accounted for 46% of fatal falls among older adults.

* Most fractures among older adults are caused by falls; the most common are fractures of the spine, hip, forearm, leg, ankle, pelvis, upper arm, and hand.

* Many survivors, who fall even if they are not injured, develop a fear of falling. This fear may cause them to limit their activities leading to reduced mobility and loss of physical fitness, which in turn increases their actual risk of falling.

At Risk?

* Men are more likely than women to die from a fall.

* Older whites are 2.5 times more likely to die from falls as their black counterparts.

* Rates also differ by ethnicity. Older non-Hispanics have higher fatal fall rates than Hispanics.

* Women are more likely than men to be injured in a fall. Women are more likely than men to suffer a non-fatal fall injury.

* Rates of fall-related fractures among older women are more than twice those for men.

* Over 90% of hip fractures are caused by falls. In 2007, there were 264,000 hip fractures and the rate for women was almost three times the rate for men.

#2 Wheelchair Transfers

Consult your psychical therapist on learning the steps for the safe wheelchair transfers you will need after returning home.

1. Wheelchair to a chair or couch.
2. Wheelchair to toilet.
3. Wheelchair to bed.
4. Wheelchair to shower bench.
5. Wheelchair to car.
6. Wheelchair to scooter.

When returning home after a stroke it will be important to be able to move from one place to another safely. This process is referred to as a 'transfer'. If you have returned home in a wheelchair like I did, you will need to learn how to move yourself from one area of your home to another in a safe manner. During any given day you will need to transfer from a wheelchair to the bed. From the bed in the morning back to the wheelchair, then let's say, from the wheelchair to the couch to watch TV. Then you will need to be able to go from the chair or couch to the toilet. That will be four to five transfers needed in the first few hours after awakening every morning.

As you can see it will be important to make many transfers every day. The more practice you have and the attention given to good form will determine you being safe in the many transfers you will have to make every day, remember that you are responsible for the lion's share of your own safety. Transfers are inherently dangerous, so be slow and deliberate in your transfers. A slip and fall could land you back in the hospital.

What makes for a safe transfer?

When transferring from a wheelchair to another location.

* Select a chair or other furniture with arm rests.

* Position yourself in the wheelchair in front of and facing where you plan to transfer to.

* Open or remove foot rests from wheelchair and lock both wheel brakes!! (Very important).

* Place both feet on the floor, shoulder width apart.

* Place strong hand on strong side wheelchair arm rest. If you have the use of both hands, place other hand on weak side wheelchair arm rest.

* Now you are set up to stand. In one fluid motion, slowly and deliberately, lean in a forward rolling motion while pushing up with one or both hands and driving yourself upward by straightening both of your legs. Stand for a few seconds and hold on firmly to the wheelchair and steady

yourself to safely stand.

* When you are steady and you have your balance turn around with your back to the intended transfer location. With small steady steps back up so the backs of both legs are up against the transfer location.

* With lower legs backed up against transfer location move strong hand from wheelchair across to strong side of the chair or other transfer location you are moving to.

* To complete the transfer, make sure to look around to see where you are going to sit. Make sure the area is clear and level. Never sit without first looking to see that it is safe to sit.

* Now with the help of your strong arm, slowly lower yourself onto the new transfer location. Never drop down uncontrolled, this could cause you to slip off a chair onto the floor and cause an unneeded injury. Always sit down in a slow controlled manner. Never transfer in a hurry.

Transferring to an automobile:

The front seat of a mid to large four-door sedan makes for a good choice when riding and transferring into a car. I have found most backseats in almost all cars to be difficult to access for the disabled.

Transfers into an automobile are much the same as other transfers. The differences may vary. To insure your safety it is important to plan ahead in choosing a car that is not too high or cramped. Pickup trucks and SUV type automobiles may have passenger seats too high for safely accessing.

Mid-size four door sedans works very well. As you get more experienced in your car transfers you will be able to ride in a larger variety of automobiles.

The car transfer:

1. Make sure the passenger door is opened all the way. Make sure the seat and floorboards are clear of all derbies that could hinder your entering the car safely.

2. Position your wheelchair directly across and facing the car seat and fully opened passenger door. Leave two feet between the car door frame and your wheelchair. Make sure

to lock both wheels of your wheelchair.

3. Now similar to your other transfers, stand up safely. Use your strong arm to steady yourself and turn around to have your back to the car. Back up to have your lower legs against the car door frame.

4. Now look around to see where you plan to sit. Never sit without looking first. You should now be in position to complete the transfer. With the help of your strong arm, reach down onto the car seat you plan to transfer to and slowly lower yourself down into the car seat.

5. Once you are safely seated bring both legs into the car. If the car has a handle located on the inside roof of the car, you can use it to help adjust yourself into the car seat.

6. You may require help with the seatbelt, if so ask the driver to assist you in buckling the seatbelt.

Dressing and personal care:

Assisting in your dressing and personal care will help to build your self-esteem and self-worth. Either totally on your own, or with the help from another family member or caregiver, these activities can help to gauge your recovery process.

If you are working with an occupational therapist, they will be the one to help you learn the steps for dressing yourself and also to get you started back to doing your personal care after a stroke.

Instruction for both these subjects can be found in "stroke hope awareness" in chapter "taking charge after a stroke".

Completing these activities is a great way of showing your loved ones that you are getting stronger and more independent.

If a caregiver helps you with these activities, find out where you are able to help and assist where you can. Remember you have the rest of your life to be able to learn to care for yourself after your stroke.

Either you or someone helping you can write down the steps needed to dress yourself. You can practice the steps, and the process will get easier and faster with time. I have detailed the steps in this resource. They are also helpful for caregivers or family to use in assisting you to obtaining a complete recovery after stroke.

Eating safely after stroke:

After fall prevention, being able to feed yourself safely is very important. After a stroke, the choking danger is a real concern for thousands of stroke survivors.

A speech therapist will work with you to develop strategies for eating safely. You should be evaluated early on to assess any limitations in diet and any other difficulties in swallowing food safely.

The loss of your ability to judge for yourself when your mouth is full can be a danger to the new stroke survivor.

After a stroke, the tongue, cheek, and throat muscles may have become lazy and unresponsive, and leave the survivor at increased danger for a choking risk.

A speech therapist will work with you on chewing, swallowing, and to judge how much food to put in your mouth at any given time.

I call it the "stroke shovel", I would have food falling out of my mouth and I would still try to put more in my already overflowing mouth, and then unable to swallow the food I was forced to spit it out and start over.

After you return home, a good place to start would be: decide which foods you can safely consume. Soft non fibrous foods are good choices to start with. Making a list like the one I made below is helpful and will give you a chance to get involved in planning your meals.

Your speech therapist would also be helpful in planning meals that are safe to eat and at the same time healthy for you. I lost 75lbs after my stroke; weight loss should be monitored after stroke by your recovery team to ensure you maintain a healthy weight.

When you find a type food that you both enjoy and is easy to swallow, you should add it to your list. This process takes some experimentation on your part, this is another chance for you to get involved in your own post stroke recovery. To ever fully rejoin the human race you must be able to eat on your own and feed yourself in a safe manner.

On your list you should try to have 10-12 food items and then you can divide them to make up three meals, breakfast, lunch, and supper.

You may be put on "liquid thickeners" for a while after a stroke. If this is the case avoid clear liquids to keep from having a choke or strangle risk.

Foods that I found to be easy to consume:

* Breakfast: Poached egg and corned beef hash, soft scrambled egg and crisp bacon. Poached egg w/butter or boiled grits. Cream of wheat, cooked oats. Yogurt w/cottage cheese. Cottage cheese w/canned peaches. Coffee, juice, and milk, thickened if needed.

* Lunch: Chicken noodle or tomato soup. Soft potato salad, mashed potatoes w/gravy. Macaroni and cheese. Grilled cheese sandwich cut up. Hamburger steak cut up. Ice cream. Protein shake, ice tee, or milk, thickened if needed. Taco meat w/ cheese and sauce.

* Supper: Mashed potatoes and gravy. Cottage cheese. Chopped spaghetti or lasagna. Chopped minute steak. Chopped canned green beans. Mild chili and boiled beans. Corn bread w/honey and butter. Peach cobbler w/ ice cream. Chopped canned pears. Protein shake, coffee, ice tea, "ensure" supplement drink, thickened if needed,

These are just some of the dishes I found I could eat after my stroke. If you take note of the foods you both like and are able to eat safely, you can mix and match to make up a menu that is tasty and safe to eat.

Easy to drink: Orange juice w/pulp. Protein shakes. Shakes, malts, thickened drinks.

Foods to use caution with or to avoid altogether: most breads. Lettuce and other raw vegetables. Undercooked meats, Chips, and French fries. Un-thickened liquids.

Many stroke survivors will be able to return home after some weeks of rehab, whereas others will need to be transferred to a full or assisted care facility. These full time care rehab facilities can run as high as $2.000 a day, like the brain injury hospital that I was able to spend a year at after my stroke. This type of care may not be available to all stroke survivors due to insurance limitations.

These facilities offer a wide range of services from rehab, minimal care, or full time nursing care if needed. Deciding on the survivors after-care requirements will depend on the level of disability caused by his or her stroke. Check with your survivor's insurance company to see what is covered in the way of care giving; there are companies that provide full or part care giving. One of the most important aspects for a survivor returning home is a safe living environment that will support and promote continued stroke recovery.

If and when you are able to return home after a stroke, members of your recovery team will need to make a visit to the home you plan to return to. They may, after an in-home inspection, suggest some changes or alterations to make the home more comfortable and safe for your successful return.

Things like rearranging the furniture so you do not need to use stairs. Removing rugs or small pieces of furniture to reduce the risk of a trip and fall. Your inspector may also advise you to install grab bars, stair rails, and shower benches for the shower and bathtub.

It is advisable to plan a trial visit home before your final discharge. These visits can help you to identify problems that need to be corrected or modified in the home prior to you returning home.

Discharge Planning

Good discharge planning should start long before your discharge from the hospital or rehab facility occurs.

This discharge planning will need to take in account the following:

1. Safety assessment
2. Living environment
3. Caregiver and family support
4. Available disability entitlements
5. The scheduling of in-home or out-patient therapies to help insure the survivor's maximum post stroke recovery
6. Plan for a twenty four hour home visit before returning home permanently.

YOUR DISCHARGE PLANNER should plan for the following:

* Make sure you return to a safe and comfortable place to live.

* Determine what care, assistance, or special equipment you will need to make the transition home.

* Arrange for continued post stroke rehab or other medical services needed by the survivor weather in-home or out-patient.

* Work with your health care provider who will monitor your loved one's health and well-being.

* Help the survivor prepare for the in-home visit by helping them make a list of questions or concerns they may have at the time of their in-home visit.

Chapter 12

Safe Walking, Scooter and Power Chair Operation after Stroke

Good safe places to walk for exercise and balance practice are:

1. Uncrowned public parks and local malls.

2. At the local grocery store or market.

When walking in unknown areas make sure to scan and watch carefully to detect any trip hazards in your path.

Walking with left neglect or any other vision cuts may cause special safety concerns for being able to walk safely.

1. Safe walking

A. I walk just like I used to drive a car. Obey all the rules of the road. It is important to give right of way to those you share the sidewalks and pathways with.

B. Slow down 30%. It's much easier to adjust your intended route and you are safer when moving slower.

C. When crossing roadways from one side to the other side. Always look one hundred yards ahead in both directions and cross only when safe.

2. Crossing at stop signs or signal light:

A. Cross at well-marked and lit crossing areas.

B. Walk or scooter up to signal light and press the walk button.

C. Now maneuver yourself or scooter down to the edge of the roadway you intend to cross and cross in the center of the handicapped cutout in the sidewalk.

D. Now focus your attention across the roadway to the walk and stop signal.

E. When light changes from stop to walk, look both ways and cross at the light and exit safely on the other side of the roadway.

3. Always give right of way

A. Walk or scooter down the middle of the path you choose. Position yourself just to the right of center of your intended path. I always walk with my left foot on the center line.

B. Always slow down and look ahead to see if people are changing positions around you. Give right of way when possible. Most times it is safer to slow down or stop altogether than to try to speed up and try to dodge an upcoming person or car.

C. Remember, if you suffer from neglect or other vision issues that restrict your sight, you are effectively blind within these vision cuts. You must exercise extra caution when walking or the operation of a motor driven scooter or power chair in public.

D. If you tire easily when walking for exercise, pick a place with places to sit and rest when you tire. Locations with places to rest may include the local mall, local and city parks, Wal-Mart, city, and federal buildings.

F. When walking out in public, try if possible to walk with your back straight and head held high. This will not only help you to see better it will give you a better appearance to the public in general. You will appear more focused and alert. People may take you more seriously and be more attentive towards you when dealing with you if you look more alert.

G. Wear sunscreen or a hat if you plan to be out in direct sun for an extended period of time.

Important side notes to remember:

1. Try to remember that it is your responsibility to practice due care when out in public places and among other people.

3. Whenever changing positions stop, look, and listen before making your move.

Indoor malls found in most areas and grocery stores are air conditioned in the summer, and many are all year around. Mobility training may include learning to use walking aids, such as a walker or cane, or a plastic brace to stabilize and assist ankle strength to help support your body's weight while you relearn how to walk.

Some therapies that may be helpful:

* Range of motion therapy uses exercises and other treatments to help lessen muscle tension (spasticity) and regain range of motion in the affected limbs.

* Psychological evaluation may involve testing your cognitive skills, counseling with a mental health professional, participating in support groups, and using medicines for mood if needed.

* Constraint-induced therapy, also known as "forced-use" therapy, involves restricting use of an unaffected limb while you practice moving the affected limb. Forcing you to use the affected arm or leg can help improve its function.

* Electrical stimulation involves using electricity to stimulate weakened muscles, causing them to contract. This may help with muscle re-education in some individuals.

* Robotic technology uses robotic devices to assist impaired limbs with performing repetitive motions, helping them regain strength and function.

* Virtual reality is an emerging, computer-based therapy that involves interacting with a simulated, real-time environment.

Chapter 13

Stroke Awareness and Prevention.

Stroke
Cerebrovascular disease; cva; cerebral infarction; cerebral hemorrhage; ischemic stroke; stroke - ischemic; cerebrovascular accident; stroke - hemorrhagic

A stroke happens when blood flow to a part of the brain stops. A stroke is sometimes called a "brain attack."

<u>Stroke strikes fast and so must you</u>

Signs of Stroke

F — is Face drooping — ask person to smile at you.

A- Tell person to raise both arms at once.

S- Ask person to repeat a simple sentence back to you.

T- Time is brain cell loss. Call 9-1-1 without delay if you or someone you're with has trouble with any of these tasks.

Stroke is third leading killer in the U.S., so do not call your family doctor's office; dial 9-1-1. Ems will evaluate and take necessary actions.

Stroke is the fourth cause of adult death in the U.S. just behind heart attack and cancer. With the baby boomers and adult obesity, it's just a matter of time till it reaches number one. One out of every six people on the planet will have a stroke.

To say having a stroke is life changing is a huge understatement. A stroke can leave you brain injured and paralyzed both physically and mentally. When a stroke occurs the blood flow to the brain is interrupted. If the brain does not receive adequate oxygen in time, the part of the brain that is affected may die and cause the body to not be able to perform normal functions. Physical therapy and rehab can in some cases result in gains of both mobility and range of motion.

Types of Strokes:

One in three smokers will suffer a stroke in their lifetime.

A stroke disrupts the flow of blood through your brain and damages brain tissue. There are two chief types of stroke. The most common type—ischemic stroke—results from blockage in an artery. The other type—hemorrhagic stroke—occurs when a blood vessel leaks or bursts. A transient ischemic attack (tia)—sometimes called a ministroke temporarily disrupts blood flow through your brain.

Ischemic stroke almost 90 percent of all strokes are ischemic strokes. They occur when the arteries to your brain are narrowed or blocked, causing severely reduced blood flow (ischemia). Lack of blood flow, cells may begin to die within minutes. The most common ischemic strokes are:

Thrombotic stroke. This type of stroke occurs when a blood clot forms in one of the arteries that supply blood to your brain. A clot usually forms in areas damaged by a disease in which the arteries are clogged by fatty deposits (plaques). This process can occur within one of the two carotid arteries of your neck that carry blood to your brain, as well as in other arteries of the neck or brain.

Embolic stroke. An embolic stroke occurs when a blood clot or other debris forms in a blood vessel away from your brain—commonly in your heart—and is swept through your bloodstream to lodge in the narrower brain arteries. This type of blood clot is called an embolus. It's often caused by irregular beating in the heart's two upper chambers (Atrial fibrillation). This abnormal heart rhythm can lead to pooling of blood in the heart and the formation of blood clots that travel elsewhere in the body.

The stroke I suffered was an embolic stroke caused by a piece of my heart valve that broke loose in my heart and traveled to my brain.

Hemorrhagic stroke hemorrhage is the medical term for bleeding. Hemorrhagic stroke occurs when a blood vessel in your brain leaks or ruptures. Brain hemorrhages can result from a number of conditions that affect your blood vessels, including uncontrolled high blood pressure (hypertension) and weak spots in your blood vessel walls (aneurysms).

Intracerebral hemorrhage. In this type of stroke, a blood vessel in the brain bursts and spills into the surrounding brain tissue, damaging cells. Brain cells beyond the leak are deprived of blood and are also damaged. High blood pressure is the most common cause of this type of hemorrhagic stroke. Over time, high blood pressure can cause small arteries inside your brain to become brittle and susceptible to cracking and rupture.

Subarachnoid hemorrhage. In this type of stroke, bleeding starts in an artery on or near the surface of the brain and spills into the space between the surface of your brain and your skull. This bleeding is often signaled by a sudden, severe "thunderclap" headache. This type of stroke is commonly caused by the rupture of an aneurysm, which can develop with age or be present from birth. After the hemorrhage, the blood vessels in your brain may widen and narrow erratically (vasospasm), causing brain cell damage by further limiting blood flow to parts of your brain.

Conditions that may put you at risk of stroke:

Long term untreated a fib can damage the heart leading to heart failure.

Atherosclerosis: also known as stroke condition. A buildup of plaque and fatty deposits in the arteries can raise your blood pressure. This plaque and fat can clog arteries and block the flow of oxygen rich blood to the brain or other parts of the body and can put you at increased risk of stroke or heart disease.

Uncontrollable risk factors:

1. Age: stroke is no respecter of age, stroke can happen to anyone. The risk of stroke increases with age. The risk doubles

after the age of 55.

2. Gender:

If you or a loved one thinks you are having, or have recently had a mini stroke, get yourself immediately to a doctor or emergency room for a complete check up to see what can be done to prevent the chance of having a future stroke.

If you should develop a "stroke condition" or are at high risk of a stroke like heart valve prolapse, narrowing arteries, coronary disease, and high blood pressure. Take the opportunity to change your life style to reduce your chance of death or disability of stroke or heart disease.

You may need to get on blood thinners, lower your cholesterol and blood pressure, and get on a low fat diet. Or in extreme cases you may even require emergency surgery to address an underlying stroke risk.

So if you think you are having any kind of stroke, mini or otherwise, don't wait, time is of the essence, act fast and get medical care immediately.

Stroke survivors, even if they escape severe mental impairment are less likely to be independent following a stroke.

Stroke survivors who were severely depressed, older, and had other health problems were more likely to be dependent than those who were younger, free of other health problems, or not depressed.

Post-stroke depression is a common problem. About 795,000 people in the United States have a stroke each year, and one-third of survivors develop depression as a result.

Even if the treatment and improvement of post-stroke depression does not directly influence recovery, it is extremely important for depression to be identified and treated, since it is associated with other health and social problems,

Transient ischemic attack (TIA)

A transient ischemic attack (TIA) or mini stroke – is a brief episode of symptoms similar to those you'd have in a stroke. The cause of a TIA is a temporary decrease in blood supply to part of your brain. Many TIAs last less than five minutes.

Like an ischemic stroke, a TIA occurs when a clot or debris blocks blood flow to part of your brain. But unlike a stroke, which involves a more prolonged lack of blood supply and causes permanent brain damage, a TIA doesn't leave lasting effects because the blockage is temporary.

Seek emergency care even if your symptoms seem to clear up. If you've had a TIA, it means there's likely a partially blocked or narrowed artery leading to your brain putting you at a greater risk of a full-blown stroke that could cause permanent damage later. And it's not possible to tell if you're having a stroke or a TIA based only on your symptoms. Up to half of those whose symptoms appear to go away are actually having a stroke that's causing brain damage.

(Mini stroke)

Mini strokes can be an important warning sign of what is to come. If you are lucky enough to get a warning before you suffer a large stroke, consider yourself fortunate. I was on the other hand not so lucky.

My stroke was caused by a blood disease that caused a piece of my heart valve to break free and get stuck in my brain and cause a major stroke resulting in some significant brain damage. I remain to this day partially blind and mostly paralyzed on my left side.

You will hear stories from well-meaning people about people they know who have suffered strokes and are completely recovered and back to work, even playing tennis and golf again. I will guarantee you that they did not have a large or more serious stroke. They most likely had a "mini stroke".

Stroke prevention:. People who used to lead independent lives before their stroke, and now must rely on outside help –

the stroke survivor will have a lot of adjusting to do — both psychologically and in the practical aspects of their day-to-day life. Therapy may help people regain more of their independence after a stroke.

Depression and suicide risk after stroke:

The risk of suicide appears to decline with time after a stroke, being greatest within the first five years following a stroke.

I would say that when you lose your fear in dying, you become at a high risk for suicide. We as "stroke survivors" can wake up after a stroke and find our whole life as we knew it erased and all the things we knew and loved are gone — our work, independence, sex, travel, food, and other pleasures we had enjoyed before stroke. It is important to try to get some of the normalcy that we knew before stroke back in our lives.

Stroke causes, and risk factors:

If blood flow is stopped for longer than a few seconds, the brain cannot get blood and oxygen. Brain cells can begin to die, causing permanent brain damage.

There are two major types of stroke: ischemic stroke and hemorrhagic stroke.

Symptoms:

The symptoms of stroke depend on what part of the brain is damaged. In some cases, a person may not know that he or she has had a stroke.

Symptoms usually develop suddenly and without warning. Or symptoms may occur on and off for the first day or two. Symptoms are usually most severe when the stroke first happens, but they may slowly get worse.

A headache may occur, especially if the stroke is caused by bleeding in the brain. The headache starts suddenly and may be severe.

Headache may occur when you are lying flat.

Wakes you up from sleep.

Gets worse when you change positions or when you bend, strain, or cough.

Other symptoms depend on how severe the stroke is and what part of the brain is affected. Symptoms may include:

Change in alertness (including sleepiness, unconsciousness, and coma).

Changes in hearing.

Changes in taste.

Changes that affect touch and the ability to feel pain, pressure, or different temperatures.

Clumsiness.

Confusion or loss of memory.

Difficulty swallowing.

Difficulty writing or reading.

Dizziness or abnormal feeling of movement (vertigo).

Lack of control over the bladder or bowels.

Loss of balance.

Loss of coordination.

Muscle weakness in the face, arm, or leg (usually just on one side).

Numbness or tingling on one side of the body.

Personality, mood, or emotional changes.

Problems with eyesight, including decreased vision, double vision, or total loss of vision.

Trouble speaking or understanding others who are speaking.

Trouble walking.

Signs and tests:

A complete exam should be done. Your doctor will:

Check for problems with vision, movement, feeling, reflexes, understanding, and speaking. Your doctor and nurses will repeat this exam over time to see if your stroke is getting worse or improving.

My stroke happened on 7/21/2006. On 4/11/2005 i was broadsided by a car that ran a red light resulting in an injury to my neck.

On 5/31/06 I started treatment for my injury. I went to a local orthopedic group for diagnosis and treatment for my injury 5/31/06. I was given pain medication and scheduled for physical therapy and an MRI on 6/3/05. When the MRI was read it showed ruptured discs at c-6 and c-7. I was then scheduled for surgery. First at ST. Jude hospital then I was changed to Fullerton surgery center where they did my "spinal fusion" as an outpatient. On 1/31/06 a doctor who worked with the orthopedic group notified my wife and I and informed them that our insurance would not cover the procedure at an outpatient center, but they proceeded anyway.

They were having difficulty with me in the recovery room but released me anyway after five hours. It was terrible. I was just about kicked out the door. I now realized that I should have listened to my brother-in-law, Jim Goatcher, and have received a second opinion from a neuro surgeon. I got home and that night had to swallow medications. They did the surgery through my mouth for goodness sakes. And five hours later I'm home in my bedroom.

Three to four months following surgery. I started experiencing severe night sweats, chills, and low grade fever with moderate to severe low back pain. I was prescribed more pain medications.

Two days before my stroke on 7/17/06 i was seen by a doctor at the orthopedic group where right in front of him I had an episode of sweats and racking chills. He did nothing and prescribed more pain medication. He did not offer any advice and I was not told to consult my family doctor. They later said that they did not take my temperature, but I know they did. Butchers, I wish I could tell you their name.

On 2/21/06 I was rushed by ambulance to ST. Jude hospital. Where it was determined by the following tests, CAT scan, EEG, and others that I had suffered a massive stroke to the right side of my brain, indirectly caused by the blood disease Endocarditis.

The blockage was caused by the vegetative state of my mitro valve. The infectious control doctor at ST. Jude ran tests and stated it was a staph infection. My cardiologist doctor at ST. Jude explained to my wife and I that I had a mitral prolapse. It was explained to me that your mitro valve, the one in the left side of your heart has leaflets that look like the tentacles on a sea anemone. When Endocarditis attacks the heart valve they call the damage it causes, a "vegetative state". We were also told that my heart was damaged beyond repair and that one day soon I would need a new heart valve/ mitro valve. It would require open heart surgery to replace it.

I had had no dental work or any other medical procedures other than the spinal fusion. There was no other source that I could have contracted the Endocarditis from. The infectious doctor put me through a six week course of intravenous antibiotics to kill the infection in my blood.

On 9/5/06 I was deemed to be infection free and was soon transferred to a rehab facility in Pomona California. I was going to be living at the tlc unit, or the transitional care unit. It was located on the hospital grounds.

My back pain continued and got increasingly more painful as time went on. I was unable to get through the sessions with my occupational therapy and especially physical therapy. This was relayed to my rehab doctor. He did an emergency MRI. When those tests had been completed and read, I was sent by ambulance to "valley community" hospital a few miles away from the rehab facility on 9/25/06. When I arrived there I was quickly admitted. There they started a series of tests. They ordered blood tests and a lumbar disc biopsy. They found I had a staph infection in the disc in my spine. I was treated with strong antibiotics once again. They thought I got the "staph" infection when I had received several blood transfusions at ST. Jude hospital while being treated for anemia. The chief of infectious diseases at Casa Colina told me he thought that my infection could have only come from the spinal fusion surgery. He thought there was no other way for it to have been introduced into my system since blood is cleaned and sterilized.

Am I at risk for a stroke? Stroke risk factors: anyone can have a stroke no matter your age, race, or gender. But, the chances of having a stroke increase if a person has certain risk factors, or conditions that can cause a stroke. The good news is that up to 80 percent of strokes can be prevented, and the best way to protect yourself and loved ones from stroke is to understand your personal risk and how to manage those stroke risks.

There are 2 types of risk factors for stroke: controllable and uncontrollable. Controllable risk factors generally fall into two categories: lifestyle risk factors, or medical risk factors. Lifestyle risk factors can often be changed, while medical risk factors can usually be treated. Both types can be managed best by working with a doctor who can prescribe medications and advise you on how to adopt a healthy lifestyle. Uncontrollable risk factors include being over the age of 55, being male, being afro-American, Hispanic or Asian/pacific islander, or having a family history of stroke or transient ischemic attack (TIA).

Controllable risk factors:
High blood pressure
Atrial fibrillation
High cholesterol
Diabetes
Atherosclerosis
Circulation problems
Tobacco use and smoking
Alcohol use
Physical inactivity
Obesity
Uncontrollable risk factors:
Age
Gender
Race
Family history
Previous stroke or TIA

(Hole in the heart)

Up to 80 percent of all strokes may be prevented — start reducing your risk now.

Although stroke can happen to anyone, certain risk factors can increase chances of a stroke. However, studies show that up to 80 percent of strokes can be prevented by working with a healthcare professional. It is important to manage personal risk and know how to recognize stroke symptoms.

The following stroke prevention guidelines will help you learn how you may be able to lower your risk for a first stroke.

High blood pressure is a major stroke risk factor if left untreated. Have blood pressure checked yearly by a doctor,at health fairs, a local pharmacy, supermarket, or with an automatic blood pressure machine.

Afib is an abnormal heartbeat that can increase stroke risk by 500%. Afib can cause blood to pool in the heart and may form a clot and cause a stroke. A doctor must diagnose and treat afib.

Smoking doubles the risk of stroke. It damages blood vessel walls, speeds up artery clogging, raises blood pressure, and makes the heart work harder.

Alcohol use has been linked to stroke in many studies. Most doctors recommend not drinking or drinking only in moderation no more than two drinks each day.

Cholesterol is a fatty substance in blood that is made by the body. It also comes in food. High cholesterol levels can clog arteries and cause a stroke. See a doctor if your total cholesterol level is more than 200.

Many people with diabetes have health problems that are also stroke risk factors. A doctor and dietician can help manage diabetes.

Excess weight strains the circulatory system. Exercise five times a week. Maintain a diet low in calories, salt, saturated and trans- fats, and cholesterol. Eat five servings of fruits and vegetables daily.

Fatty deposits can block arteries carrying blood to the

brain and lead to a stroke. Other problems such as sickle cell disease or severe anemia should be treated.

A TIA is a temporary episode of stroke-like symptoms that can last a few minutes to 24 hours but usually causes no permanent damage or disability. Tia and stroke symptoms are the same. Recognizing and treating a TIA can reduce your stroke risk. Up to 40 percent of people who experience a TIA may go on to have a stroke.

The relation between acute ischemic stroke and infection is complex. Infection appears to be an important trigger that proceeds up to a third of ischemic strokes and can bring about stroke through a range of potential causes.

Before teeth cleaning or any type of evasive surgery, play it safe and take antibiotics before and after the procedure. I had afib and had a spinal fusion, and four months later suffered a massive stroke caused by Endocarditis, a blood infection.

What is drop foot?

With regards to drop foot; in relation to stroke. When someone is paralyzed in the leg, foot, or ankle, if you lose control of the foot, toes, and ankle you run the risk of developing the condition known as "drop foot".

When I was in the hospital after my stroke I was given boots designed to help control the onset of "drop foot". When brain injury is such that you lose the use of your ankle and toes, you are more apt to develop "drop foot". I wear an a.f.o. because I have lost all use of my left ankle. Without the use of the a.f.o, I am at a high risk of falling, due to me dragging my toes when I walk.

On braces for patients with drop foot:

Drop foot is a term that describes a disorder where a survivor has a limited ability or inability to raise the foot at the ankle joint. This makes walking difficult, as the toes tend to drag on the ground which leads to tripping and instability. Patients adapt to this by using their hip muscles to exaggerate lifting the foot above the ground or by swinging their leg outward so that the foot can clear the ground.

Drop foot is often treated with the use of braces. The goal of bracing is to provide patients with a more normal and comfortable gait. Drop foot can be treated with several different types of braces. Deciding on which brace to use depends on each survivor's individual condition. When treating drop foot, afos can act in several different ways to help the survivor.

To understand how afos work, you must first understand two standard motions that occur at the ankle joint or dorsiflexion and plantarflexion. Plantarflexion is the motion the ankle joint makes when the toes point downward. Dorsiflexion is the motion the ankle joint makes when the foot points upward. This motion needs to occur when the foot comes off the ground so that the patient does not drag their toes. Patients with drop foot usually have a partial or complete weakness of the muscles that flex the foot at the ankle joint.

You can use several different types of afos to treat drop foot in stroke survivors. Some of them are custom and require a mold be made of your foot, ankle, and leg. Others are prefabricated. The goal is to provide patients with a comfortable afo that will give them the best fit and support.

A quick way to test for drop foot is to try to walk on the heels. If this proves difficult, drop foot may be present.

In order to pursue appropriate drop foot treatment a specialist in this field should be consulted.

Preventing falls is very important for stroke patients.

People who have had a stroke fall almost three times more often as people who haven't had a stroke.

In a study of 1,104 stroke survivors, 40 percent reported at least one fall during the first six months after their stroke. Of the 407 participants who fell, 35 percent sustained an injury that required medical treatment and 10 percent sustained a fracture.

Researchers also found:

Older aged survivors, a prior fall, previous stroke, prior dependency before stroke, poor cognitive status, and low mood such as depression were associated with a higher risk of falls or falls with injury after stroke.

Women were more likely to sustain injury from a fall than men.

Those survivors who fell in the year prior to stroke were 2x times more likely to fall after stroke.

Stroke survivors who were more dependent were twice as likely to fall after stroke.

Those with higher levels of functioning were 80 percent less likely to sustain injury after stroke.

Those who were depressed were almost 2x times as likely to fall as those who weren't.

We need to increase the awareness among family members on fall prevention. More than one-third of stroke survivors will fall after a stroke and the consequences can be disastrous.

There will come a time after "stroke" when you will tell yourself, "I can walk without my cane or walker". Don't do it unless you have been cleared by a certified physical therapist to walk without an aid. You run a high risk of having a fall. Brain injury and even death are a constant threat to stroke survivors after stroke. I made the mistake recently myself and have broken my hand and wrist in a fall.

My fall:

On 7/09/12, while going from the couch to the coffee pot in the kitchen at my home. A trip I had made a thousand times since returning home after my stroke. I lost my balance, and when I started to fall over, I was unable to stop myself from falling.

I fell to my weak side and landed with the full weight of my body on my left hand and wrist. Before I knew it, I had severely fractured my left hand and wrist. Like old men do, who are too stubborn to go to the doctor or call 911 when they have chest pain and then die from a heart attack, I also refused to go in and get checked out after my fall.

I started self-medicating myself with pain killers I had on hand. I foolishly thought that if I waited a few days it would quit hurting and just go away. After all, it was my paralyzed arm; I could not use it anyway.

Unfortunately that is a common way of thinking for stroke survivors. But nothing is further from the truth. Many serious conditions can develop from untreated injuries. It's better to error on the side of caution. You not only put your overall health at risk but put undue concern and worry on those who care for you.

If you take a fall and think you have injured yourself, do not wait! Tell a caregiver, spouse, or call 911 immediately, especially if you have struck your head in a fall. You may not experience pain after a fall, but you could have underlying injuries that could become life threatening. Bleeding to the brain does not always cause significant pain, and could end up being fatal if gone untreated. Never, and I stress never — walk without a walking aid, (cane or walker) or get out of your wheelchair unless you have doctor's orders to do so.

I waited a full week to go to the doctors, had I waited two more days I was told, I would not be able to have the fractures to my hand and wrist set and placed in a cast to insure them healing properly. The attending orthopedic doctor told me if I had missed the ten day cutoff period, my hand and wrist may have healed crooked and I would most likely have to have had surgery to ever get them to heal correctly.

A common misconception of stroke survivors is that, "if I hurt myself on one of my "weak" or paralyzed limbs, it doesn't matter", they cannot use them anyway. If you think you have been injured by a fall, there is a very good chance you have been! Once again, after a fall make sure to be checked out and do not wait!

As a result of my stroke, I suffer from both of these conditions:

Hemiplegia is total paralysis of the arm, leg, and/ or trunk on the same side of the body. Hemiplegia is more severe than hemiparesis, wherein one half of the body has less marked weakness. Hemiplegia may be congenital or acquired from an illness or stroke.

Hemiplegia is not an uncommon medical disorder. In elderly individuals, strokes are the most common cause of hemiplegia. In children, the majority of cases of hemiplegia has no identifiable cause and occurs with a frequency of about one in every thousand births. Experts indicate that the majority of cases of hemiplegia that occur up to the age of two should be considered to be cerebral palsy until proven otherwise.

Left neglect hemispatial neglect is most frequently associated with left neglect.

Hemi-pelagic and Left-neglect syndrome is a neuropsychological condition in which, after damage to one hemisphere of the brain, a deficit in attention to and awareness of one side of space is observed. It is defined by the inability for a person to process and perceive stimuli on one side of the body or environment that is not due to a lack of sensation. Hemispatial neglect is very commonly related to the damaged hemisphere of the brain, but instances of ipsilesional neglect (on the same side as the lesion) have been reported.

Hemispatial neglect results most commonly from brain injury to the right cerebral hemisphere, causing visual neglect of the left-hand side of space. Right-sided spatial neglect is rare because there is redundant processing of the right space by both the left and right cerebral hemispheres, whereas in most left-dominant brains the left space is only processed by the right cerebral hemisphere. Although most strikingly affecting visual perception ('visual neglect'), neglect in other forms of perception can also be found—either alone, or in combination with visual neglect.

For example, a stroke affecting the right parietal lobe of

the brain can lead to neglect for the left side of the visual field, causing a patient with neglect to behave as if the left side of sensory space is nonexistent (although they can still turn left). In an extreme case, a patient with neglect might fail to eat the food on the left half of their plate, even though they complain of being hungry. If someone with neglect is asked to draw a clock, their drawing might show only numbers 12 to 6, or all 12 numbers on one half of the clock face, the other side being distorted or left blank. Neglect patients may also ignore the weak side of their body, shaving or adding make-up only to the non-neglected side. These patients may frequently collide with objects or structures such as door frames on the side being neglected.

Neglect may also present as a delusional form, where the patient denies ownership of a limb or an entire side of the body. Since this delusion often occurs alone without the accompaniment of other delusions, it is often labeled as a monothematic delusion.

Neglect not only affects present sensation but memory and recall perception as well. A patient suffering from neglect may also, when asked to recall a memory of a certain object and then draw said object, again, only draw half of the object. It is unclear; however, if this is due to a perceptive deficit of the memory (having lost pieces of spatial information of the memory) or whether the information within the memory is whole and intact, but simply being ignored, the same way portions of a physical object in the patient's presence would be ignored. This is the kind of left-neglect that I suffer from, due to a stroke I suffered and the resulting brain injury to the right side of my brain.

We who have lived through a stroke prefer "survivor" to victim. We are most assuredly victims to a terrible event in our lives, but more importantly we are survivors.

When dealing with a stroke survivor, refer to their effected limbs as "weak" or "strong" rather than "good" or "bad". Just because they do not have use of an arm or leg, that does not make that limb "bad".

Chapter 14

Subluxation, Tone & Botox after Stroke

This section deals with the conditions that may occur in some individuals after a stroke

1. Subluxation:

What is a shoulder subluxation?

A shoulder subluxation is a temporary or partial dislocation of the shoulder joint. The shoulder is a ball and socket joint. The ball of the upper arm bone (humorous) is held into the socket of the shoulder blade (scapula) by a group of ligaments.

How does it occur?

A shoulder subluxation can occur from falls onto your outstretched arm, direct blows to your shoulder, or having your arm forced into an awkward position. If you have had a previous injury or if your shoulder ligaments are naturally loose, you may sublux your shoulder doing simple activities like throwing or putting on a shirt or jacket.

Symptoms of a shoulder subluxation include:

* The feeling that your shoulder has gone "in and out of joint"

* Looseness in your shoulder

* Pain, weakness, or numbness in your shoulder or arm

Your doctor will talk to you about your symptoms and perform a physical exam. Many times the diagnosis of a shoulder subluxation is made by your description of the injury. When your doctor examines you, they may find that your shoulder is loose and may partially slip out of joint during the exam. Your doctor may order x-rays to see if you have had any fractures.

The pain from a shoulder subluxation is treated with ice packs for 20 to 30 minutes, 3 to 4 times a day. You may take an anti-inflammatory medication. You may need to avoid painful activities until the pain improves.

The most important treatment for the looseness in the shoulder that causes a subluxation is shoulder strengthening exercises. Shoulders that continue to sublux and cause painful symptoms may require surgery to correct the joint looseness.

Subluxation is common in the shoulder joints of the weak side arm or arms of stroke survivors after stroke. When loss of muscle occurs, the weight of the arm creates a constant pulling affect against the shoulder joint. This can cause a slow dislocation of the arm from the ball socket of the shoulder joint.

When sitting, walking, or laying support your arm weight to reduce chances of developing subluxation.

Exercises and preventive steps to help combat subluxation:

When laying down use a pillow to support the weak arm. When sitting use a pillow or sit in a chair with good wide armrests.

When spending extended time in a wheelchair be sure to use an arm tray. These can be found online or at a medical supply store.

The risk of subluxation occurring increases after a stroke.

"Subluxation" can be painful and difficult to reverse. You should start from the earliest days to identify it and take steps to reduce its causes. Whenever you are out of bed take care to support the affected arm or arms.

Prevention and Precautions:

* Doing shoulder shrugs can strengthen the back muscles and help to minimize subluxation.

* The use of a good sling can also take strain off the weight of the arm and the shoulder joint, therefore reducing the chance of subluxation.

* Always support weak limbs with pillows or an "arm

tray" when possible.

2. Tone:

What are the symptoms of dystonia, or "tone"? Tone can affect many different parts of the body. Early symptoms may include deterioration in handwriting, foot cramps, and/or a tendency of one foot to pull up or drag; this may occur "out of the blue" or may occur after running or walking some distance. The neck may turn or pull involuntarily, especially when the patient is tired or stressed. Sometimes both eyes will blink rapidly and uncontrollably, rendering a person to become functionally blind. Other possible symptoms are tremor and voice or speech difficulties. The initial symptoms can be very mild and may be noticeable only after prolonged exertion, stress, or fatigue. Over a period of time, the symptoms may become more noticeable and widespread and be unrelenting.

How are the dystonias classified?

After a stroke you may experience a condition known as "tone". It is most often found in the foot and arm and hands of stroke survivors. "Tone" in the hand and arm may cause the hand on the weak side to clench inward in a closed fist manner.

This condition should also be addressed early on after stroke when first identified. After brain injury, the body — in a protective response to brain injury — will try to return to the "fetal" position by pulling inward.

Some ways to counteract this condition:

* The use of a good hand brace. These can be purchased online, at a medical supply, or custom made; these custom braces can be very expensive.

* Botox in recent years has become a good treatment for the condition of "Tone". Injections into the affected muscles are made every three to four months or as a doctor recommends. It takes two to three weeks after injections to

take full effect.

Many insurances carriers cover Botox therapy but some do not. My injections run $1,500 every three months.

Remember individual results will vary, depending on the severity of the "Tone". I get excellent results and Botox has been a minor miracle for me. I highly recommend that anyone with "Tone" issues get advice from a doctor that has experience in the field of Botox and the condition of "Tone". I also use a good hand brace at night to help keep my affected hand in an open position. This helps to control my "Tone". If you are consistent and you wear the brace nightly, you may get good results also.

Increased "Tone" in your arm or leg, may be triggered by stroke or transient ischemic attack , i.e. TIA, "mini stroke", or any brain injury can be treated and managed to reduce the side effects of "Tone". There are effective strategies that you can apply which will significantly reduce your "Tone" and the accompanying pain, stiffness, decreased range of motion, and decreased functional use following stroke.

Apply moist heat via a hot water bottle wrapped in a towel to your arm or leg. Place the heat over the muscle or muscle group that is tight and sore. Add additional towels if your skin cannot tolerate the heat for 15 minutes.

Rub the sore and tight area of your arm or leg with moderate pressure, increasing the blood flow to the tissue. Locate the muscle or tendon that feels tight and press perpendicular to the tight fibers for up to 90 seconds until your fibers relax. Stretch out the tight joint while applying pressure.

Perform range of motion to the stiff joint to relax your muscles three to four times daily. Grab your limb below the tight area and stretch it in every direction, moving slowly and concentrating on the movement throughout. Hold your limb for 10 seconds when it is stretched out and release slowly.

Prevent a contracture by wearing a splint to your arm or leg with increased "Tone". See a physical or occupational therapist to be fitted for a splint. Wear your splint six hours per day, or while sleeping at night if your splint impedes your function.

Tips and warnings:

* When applying pressure, do not move your hand until the tendon or muscle relaxes. Use your thumb or two fingertips to apply the pressure.

* Consult your treating physician or therapist for splint recommendations. Remove splint and discontinue use if any redness or sore spots occur. Serious injury can occur with range of motion exercises for increased tone so use care when exercising. If you have severe pain when performing any of these tasks, discontinue the task immediately. Do not use moist heat if you have vascular issues or diabetes as this could burn your skin.

Things you'll need

* Splint for hand or foot.

* After stroke or any other cause of brain injury, the body wants to return to the fetal position. You will find it is much easier to complete the inward motions of arms and legs. The opening outwards of arms and the flexing outward motion of your week side may be more difficult or in my case pretty much completely impossible.

The "Tone" or muscle tightness associated with "Tone" can be lessened by the use of Botox and is intended to help elevate and lessen this condition known as "Tone". As described in the preceding article.

Botox

My experience with Botox.

It was after my time at the famous brain injury hospital Casa Colina. I had already returned home. But I still saw my rehab doctor. My hand was starting to ball up and the muscles would cramp up and stay that way for days at a time. I was told that after a stroke and brain injury that the body wanted to protect itself and return to a fetal position.

From the very beginning, following my stroke, everything that showed some promise we would try and see if there was any merit to it. Some things worked temporary, but many others showed no lasting benefit. I never forgot those conversations with accident or stroke patients I had back at the rehab facility. They raved about the new treatments they were getting. I had heard of Botox used by wealthy women to reduce age lines in their faces.

Like I said, I had returned home at this time. When I had my next appointment with Dr. Lee, my rehab doctor, I inquired about the use of Botox for the condition. I had started experiencing the condition called "Tone" and the stiffing of the muscles in my hand. He said that it couldn't hurt to check it out and referred me to a pain management doctor named Peter White, a big easy going Aussie. A Real good regular kind of guy. I have had moderate to severe "Tone" in my weak side hand. My arm and hand have remained paralyzed since 7/06, almost seven years now. I started taking Botox injections two years ago, and the Botox treatments have been a miracle for me. Not only does the Botox relax my hand to allow me to sleep better it makes me appear more normal to those I come in contact with in my daily life.

I'm sure you all can remember the old man who walked with a limp and had one of his hands drawn up into a claw-like fist or "death grip".

After stroke it is important to fit in and rejoin the human race. When, as survivors, we look handicapped, we are more likely to be treated as handicapped or less than equal.

Test a rubber arm with sensors that beep when a needle hits the proper muscle. I think it's valuable to make sure you're in the right place. Doctor White uses an ultrasound to see where to inject the Botox into my forearm.

Best known by the brand name Botox, has many medical

uses, some official and some off label. It helps dystonia victims regain control of spamming muscles, and children with clubfoot avoid surgery.

Its use in stroke victims is still off label — that is, it is not approved for that purpose by the food and drug administration. But it is so widely accepted that Medicare and other insurers will usually reimburse for its use.

Only about 5 percent of the stroke patients who could benefit from its use ever get it.

Primary care doctors who oversee nursing homes often do not know about it. Relatively few doctors are trained to do the injections, which go much deeper than dermatologists do to erase frown lines. And most neurologists are in the habit of prescribing antispasticity drugs like tizanidine and baclofen, which are oral and inexpensive, but which cause drowsiness and weaken every muscle in the body, not just the target ones.

Can Botox aid stroke victims?

November 20, 2008

Botox is considered a poison. Millions of Americans use it to help smooth their wrinkles. As more people use Botox as the ultimate wrinkle remover, doctors are realizing that its benefits go far deeper than the skin. Now it's being used to help stroke victims.

What is Botox?

Botox is a brand name for botulinum toxin type a. It's produced by the bacterium clostridium botulinum.

What does Botox do?

In 1989, long before physicians injected Botox into faces to smooth wrinkles, the FDA approved it for patients with debilitating neurological diseases such as dystonia (Tone). In these conditions, faulty connections between brain and muscle cause parts of the body to spasm. Muscles are locked into uncomfortable, often excruciating, positions. Amazingly, Botox liberated many of these patients by actually chemically allowing their muscles to relax.

This ability to stop the brain from triggering the muscle malfunction led researchers to use Botox for a whole host of other conditions. Up to four in 10 stroke survivors suffer from spastic disability. You may recognize it as stiffness on one side of the body, often seen in a club-like hand or foot. These people lose their independence — the ability to wash themselves, to eat, even walk. Botox has been used for years in these stroke patients in combination with physical therapy. It allows some of them to gain back mobility and function in their muscles.

Is Botox the perfect solution?

Botox isn't a cure-all. It can have minor side effects and more studies need to be done on long-term use. But for many patients, Botox provides the muscle relief that will allow them to better move their affected limbs.

Chapter 15

Survivor or Victim
You Make the Choice.

Stroke recovery

AS SURVIVORS "WHAT DOES NOT KILL US ONLY MAKES US STRONGER"

Webster defines victim and survivor as:

Victim. Survive

Definition of survive

1: to remain alive or in existence: to live on.

2: to continue to function or prosper.

Survive survivor

V.Sur*vived, sur*viv*ing, sur*vives

V.intr.

1. To remain alive or in existence.

2. To carry on despite hardships or trauma; persevere: families that were surviving in tents after the flood.

3. To remain functional or usable: I dropped the radio, but it survived.

V.tr.

The word victim comes from the Latin word victimia which means to sacrifice.

You will discover soon if you are not already aware, that you will be in for the fight of your life when you wake up after suffering a stroke.

Recovery after stroke will be a hard fight at best. Your stroke recovery must be taken on as an all or nothing proposition. You must start stroke recovery as early as possible after your stroke and as intensely as possible for as long as possible. This is where the rubber meets the road as they say. This is truly where I got the title for this chapter. "Survivor or victim", you ultimately will make the choice.

I have discovered through extensive research and

personal experience that there is no such thing as the proverbial "Magic bullet". It just does not exist. I have come to realize that most people think that if someone who suffered a stroke just waits around long enough it will pass like the passing of a bad cold.

Another common misconception is that the survivor is just not trying hard enough.

After stroke it is not the affected muscles that are weak but the brain that controls the muscles that is many times the cause. Unlike muscle or bone, the brain damage caused by a debilitating stroke never heals.

The gains you can get back after a stroke are in the early days following the stroke event. This could be from hours to months, rarely years.

How to get a stroke survivor to exercise

When it comes to dealing with a loved one who has had a stroke, it's never easy. There are difficulties that stand in the way, and sometimes those difficulties are from the actual person themselves because they are refusing to exercise. When a stroke survivor refuses to exercise or chooses not to exercise as much as they should be, it can be an incredibly frustrating experience. Here are some simple tips on how to get your loved one to exercise after they have had a stroke.

Encourage, encourage, encourage. There is nothing worse for a person that is in a bad situation is to get no encouragement from the people around them, especially their loved ones. If a stroke survivor is partially paralyzed, the smallest triumph deserves praise. A little encouragement and a lot of positive reinforcement can go a long way.

Give them a stress ball. After a stroke, the survivors' body has become weakened; it can be a long and arduous task to getting it back on track; so it's a good idea to start off small and simple. That little stress ball can do wonders, especially between physical therapy and/or when the person is confined to their bed or a wheel chair. Not only is the stress ball good for their hands, but it's good for the person's arm and chest muscles too. A stress ball is easily accessible to do at any time and it's small so they can keep it in their pocket and do it wherever they are.

Consider giving them small 1 lb. Weights. While it may not seem like much, after the muscles have weakened, having them use a 1 lb Weight can be quite a bit of help. There are 1 lb. ankle weights and 1 lb. arm weights which can be purchased very cheaply at the local sporting goods store or online. Give them a certain amount to do and count down with them as they finish their reps. Be there with them and cheer them on to finish.

Consult the stroke survivor's doctor and see what you can have your loved one do on their physical therapy off days to help them work out their body. Sometimes you have to ask. Make sure you ask the doctor first before having the stroke survivor do any type of exercise.

Have patience, show compassion, but exhibit tough love. You don't totally know what the stroke survivor is going through unless you've been in their shoes. However, sometimes a little tough love is needed. Your loved one may need a reminder that they need to work harder in order for them to get better, so a little kick in the butt by the people that they care about may be a big help.

What makes you a victim? You Choose to Be a Victim.

Self-love and allowing yourself to be a victim don't go together. Victims rarely love themselves. It's not respecting yourself to let others mistreat you. People will ask themselves, "Why do people abuse me? Why me? And will whine, "I'll never get what I want because I allow myself to be a victim." It's your choice to be a victim. People don't make you a victim. You allow yourself to be one.

Victims blame others. But no one can take your power away if you do not give it away!

Do you blame others for being unhappy? Do you complain that you hate being a victim? Playing a victim is a conscious choice survivors make. Nobody can force you to give up your power to make your own choices. When you take charge of your life, you become the master of your own life. Victims always complain about who did them wrong. When you act like a loser, people will treat you like a loser. After all, we usually get back what we give out.

Your response to life's trials will determine whether you are a victim or a survivor. I know it can be hard. But deciding to relinquish the victim role and stand up for yourself will attract a better treatment and increases your self-respect. Eliminate self-pity and change your situation! Do not remain a victim one more day. Taking a stand makes people less likely to take advantage of you. You have control of how people treat you. Complaining is a waste of valuable time. Nobody can abuse someone who won't stand for it, and nobody is a victim unless they choose to be. Once you stand up to people, and for yourself, you will see how much power you have. Victims feel helpless, which brings self-esteem down. But remember, you're not helpless.

You always have spiritual support in lifting yourself up from living as a victim, so pray and lean on God.

Remember that the ball is in your court. Think about what makes you feel like a victim and how you can change things that make you feel that way. The more you work on self-love, the less you'll allow people to treat you poorly. When you love yourself, you won't want to allow yourself to be a victim. Being a Nice Person is o.k. but do you accept suffering as punishment for not being good enough!

That kind of attitude destroys self-esteem! It's your choice to adopt a victim mentality or handle situations in ways that give your control back to you. Don't give away your power to others.

What makes you a survivor? There is more to survival than survival gear and skills. A survival topic not often touched upon is how personality traits of individuals affect their ability to survive in adverse conditions.

In nature's great wisdom it has created a wide variety of people, no two of which share the same exact physical and personality traits. This is good and insures the survival of the species come what may. Even misfits have their place in the world, but true survivors are typically people of action and skill.

Traits of the survivor include:
Commitment to survive when the going gets tough — the most important survival skill is contained within your mind. You need to want to survive, no matter the situation and prospect of outcome. Survivors never give up.

Curiosity and Inquisitiveness
The desire to learn and discover how things work will hone your skills in a wide variety of subjects. Play is nature's way of having you learn and develop skills in preparation for the real thing when your playful experience suddenly becomes the deciding factor in whether you make it or not.

Keep your Sense of Humor
What is known as Gallows humor has lightened the perceived load of many a survivor. Your sense of humor works as a pressure release mechanism. And if you can make light of your difficulties, you are placing yourself above them — a good position from which to take the action you may need to survive.

Deal quickly with Uncertainty
The ability to continue on through adversity, even when there is conflicting information and uncertainty. The survivor takes action when action is required, trusting that as events

unfold they can fine tune their approach and successfully achieve the desired outcome.

Get over it

The survivor mentality does not waste time pining over past mistakes or failures. Dwelling on regrets and disappointments will change nothing, and is counterproductive. The best way to survive is to learn all you can for the situation you are in, and plan future action toward your best advantage.

Be Adaptive

The successful wilderness survivor has the ability to take charge and control the environment they are in using their knowledge and only the materials at hand. They can improvise quickly to find new ways to succeed where none existed before. Whatever happens, the best survivors tackle problems head on and find solutions.

Those who practice the survival arts become a special breed of person. The personality traits of the survivor spill over into successful everyday life. Survivors meet life's challenges with confidence; they improvise, adapt, and overcome. These are people who have a view of the world that does not paint them as a victim. They tend to not be whiners who are always complaining about the bad things that are happening to them. The first thing many people do when something bad happens to them is to be in denial. People who make good survivors tend to get through that phase quickly and accept the situation they find themselves in.

The Terminator types are the first to go; many of the disaster survivors studied weren't the most skilled, strongest, or the most experienced in their group.

Those who seemed best suited for survival, the strongest or most skilled were many times the first to die off in life-or-death situations. Experience and physical strength can lead to carelessness. The terminator types are often the first to go.

Small children and inexperienced climbers, for example, often survived emergencies in the wilderness far better than their stronger or adult counterparts.

They survive because they're humble. They know when to rest, when they shouldn't try something beyond their capabilities, and know when it's wise to be afraid.

Humility can keep you out of trouble. If you go busting into the unknown with the attitude that you know everything, you run the risk of missing important clues for success.

Survivors tend to be independent thinkers as well. When hijacked planes hit the World Trade Center during the September 11, 2001, terrorist attacks, hundreds of workers were trapped in the towers. Security told many of them to stay put and wait for rescue.

Most of those who heeded the directions from security died in the burning towers. Most of the survivors decided to ignore what they were told by security and instead headed downstairs through the smoke-filled towers and did not wait to be rescued.

Survivors are not rule followers, they think for themselves and keep an independent frame of mind.

Survivors also share another trait, they have strong family bonds. Many survivors report that they are motivated to endure hardships by a desire to be with loved ones again.

Survivors also pay attention to their intuition, if something tells them that something isn't safe to do that day, they'll back off, even if they think they are able to do it at first thought.

About the Author

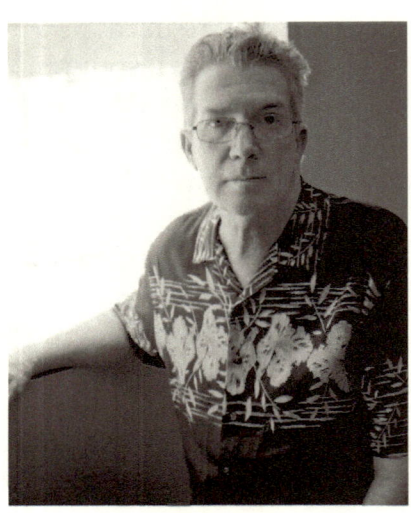

I am Daniel Bryan Jones 57 years old.

I was born in west Texas and have lived in Southern California most of my life. I am married with one grown daughter and three beautiful grandchildren. I have worked for myself since I married in 1975. I owned and operated a residential roofing company for the first twenty-five years. I retired from roofing in 1989 and spent the next ten years traveling the world's mission fields. When I finished my last mission trip to West Africa, I went into the real estate business where I became successful in selling high end properties in southern California.

I graduated high school in 1974 and have been self-taught and am a self-made man through my many business projects over the last thirty five years.

I suffered a massive stroke in 2006 that was life changing. After years of recovery I started writing. I have recently been writing the amazing story of my time in the mission field. Every story is 100% true. I am in the process of writing a three book series on stroke awareness, prevention, and recovery. In addition I am also writing a training and exercise manual for post stroke survivors. Also in the works is a guide to care giving for caregivers. And lastly, I have an autobiography on my life story half written up to 1999.

Since my stroke I have been asked to speak at many of the Southland Colleges and lecture on the effects of stroke and the awareness, prevention, and recovery of stroke. I volunteer every Monday for a stroke group that lends support to those who suffer from "aphasia", a condition caused by strokes that renders it victims unable to communicate. I had recently spoke as the key note speaker at the 2012 Survivor's Symposium, for the National Institute for Speaking and Language Association.

LINKS:

FACE BOOK: https://www.facebook.com/pages/The-Foundation-for-Stroke-Awareness-and-Recovery/115644581918230?ref=ts&fref=ts

WEBSITE:
http://www.daneilbryanjones.com